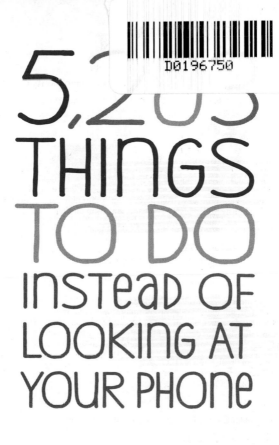

5,203 THINGS TO DO INSTEAD OF LOOKING AT YOUR PHONE

BARBARA ANN KIPFER

WORKMAN PUBLISHING · NEW YORK

DEDICATION

To Paul, Kyle, Keir, and Hoops—who give me plenty of
good things to do that do not involve any devices.

Library of Congress Control Number: 2020938552

ISBN 978-1-5235-0985-0

Design by Galen Smith

Illustrations by Scot Ritchie

Workman books are available at special discounts when purchased in
bulk for premiums and sales promotions as well as for fund-raising or
educational use. Special editions or book excerpts can also be created
to specification. For details, contact the Special Sales Director at the
address below or send an email to specialmarkets@workman.com.

Workman Publishing Co., Inc.
225 Varick Street
New York, NY 10014-4381

workman.com

WORKMAN is a registered trademark of Workman Publishing Co., Inc.

Printed in the United States

First printing August 2020

10 9 8 7 6 5 4 3 2 1

INTRODUCTION

Most of us can admit that we look at our phones or tablets more often than we need to. We use them at times when we could be making direct contact with others, with our environment, with an activity, or with the present moment. Although a lot of good comes from these devices, they also have negative effects on our attention, equilibrium, and social skills. Unplugging to reconnect, focus, and calm our minds is a never-ending opportunity.

Time spent on physical activities and sports, reading, or creating and engaging directly with others is critical to healthy physical and social development. One of my best friends is my iPad mini, but while writing this book, I started hiking, increased my biking, set up a home gym, and tried indoor climbing. I've been adding to those physical activities ever since and I feel better than ever in body and mind. I keep my little iPad friend tucked away, but I visit with her regularly—though far less often and with clearer intentions.

We'd all feel a bit better if we'd slow down, reflect, pay attention, be awake and aware, and become comfortable with silence, solitude, and unfilled time. I hope this book will remind you that your world is much more than can be seen or accessed via a screen, and that it will help you ask yourself what makes you feel nourished and grounded as a human being.

And for those of you who must have a phone on hand for one reason or another, I've suggested several ways to use your phone that are more creative and mind-expanding than scrolling on social media or playing a familiar game. They're marked with a tiny phone icon.

Enjoy getting (re)acquainted with the world outside your phone!

—Barbara Ann Kipfer

Smile at a stranger

put a bag in your car for litter

write a letter to your future self

plan a 24-hour liquid diet

notice the air on your skin

do calligraphy for a party invitation

go for a silent drive

make an accordion book

plan a beach day

visit a botanical garden

keep a journal of the most beautiful
  things you see

talk to someone who needs company

design a book cover

watch a cat drink or eat

play a board game

try a breakfast burrito

**make your backyard
inviting for wildlife**

ask a bunch of questions

make the best case you can for a point of
view that you totally oppose

solve a What's wrong with this picture?
puzzle

follow a bird's flight

come up with 10 alternate uses for an
object

peruse your adolescent belongings

create an artist's studio

explore a beach in the off-season

choose a different first name for yourself

close your eyes and study what appears

change your desk or view

make a Zen garden

check out a cute guy or girl

take the back roads

solve a brainteaser

invent a cookie

pretend to be a great artist

open a book at random and read

eat a banana slowly

play with a child

create your day in advance by thinking
about the way you want it to go

plant a butterfly garden

learn a great synonym for a word you
love or use a lot

look through a kaleidoscope

try to be a rainbow in someone's cloud

list all the berries you can think of

finish a backlog

get your car washed

find an intact shell on the beach

enjoy the aroma of a beverage before
the first sip

decide what and who you want to care
about and pay attention to

cook a meal from an unfamiliar ethnicity

decorate a box to keep your treasures in

remember to bring everything
you need

put on a puppet show

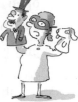

check the back of your mind to see
if there are any ideas lurking

learn 14 ways to fold a napkin

help a child find unexpected ways of
playing with household objects

complete a book proposal

use a gift someone gave you

make a wish list

write a setting for a play or story

throw away all the unhealthy food in
your cabinets

explore the attic

tell someone how great they look

drive to a beach

catch a butterfly in the palm of your hand, then let it go

put your favorite chair in front of a window

take something apart and discover just how many parts it has

write down a significant memory from each year of your life

study the behavior of someone who won't notice

walk a child to school

stop to listen to a street musician

treat yourself to a favorite food

take an aptitude test

spin a ball on your fingertip

set up a breakfast nook

go library browsing

put together a great workout

spend an hour blindfolded

put the bike rack on the car

practice a walk that projects confidence

prepare a five-course dinner

play in a sandbox

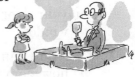

improve your attitude
toward one person or
situation in your life

pay attention to all the tiny balancing
movements your body makes as you
sit or stand

get to know a side of someone most
people don't see

fill a flask with a hot drink and share it
with someone

focus on a painting you find intriguing

observe a building site

fix a basic plumbing problem

make up a career for each person you see

design your dream something

hunt for the source of a single specific
sound

count the geese in a flying V-formation

host a clothing swap

make a "Welcome Home" banner

take a weekend retreat at a convent

wash the bedspread

have your car fixed

turn your commuting time into thinking time

go through an old box full of childhood things

throw a backyard party

give a book to someone to make them laugh

think of a question you would like answered, then look for three clues that could be the answer

admire someone's bookshelves

teach your pet a new trick

focus on hearing every sound you can for a day

sit in a café and people-watch

fill the car with gas

tell someone about a book you enjoyed

leave a dollar bill where someone will discover it

set a beautiful table for a family-only dinner

experiment with a different way to get somewhere

read the fine print on everything

dress up for dinner at home

draw on a frosty window

plan a fall leaf trip

donate an ant farm to a kindergarten

perfect your basketball layup

do your banking

participate in a beach cleanup

devise a marketing strategy

give your pet a massage

name your appliances

buy a lottery ticket

make sure all the doors are locked

build something amazing with LEGOs

make a water slide

ask questions about others' opinions

fill a basket with a blanket, a good book,
and a snack, and head for the park

ask for a back scratch or back rub

create a world of your own, wherever you
happen to be

arrange a vase of flowers

hang a "Do Not Disturb" sign up for a
while and use your office, bedroom,
porch, or yard as a refuge

spend an hour alternating between
15 minutes outside and 15 minutes
inside

go out in the woods alone and just think

allow yourself a Zen moment

give yourself a head start on something

get someone a welcome back present

fill out a timeline with your major
life events

learn to whittle

**do a face-the-wall meditation, sitting
12 to 18 inches from a completely
blank wall**

add a blanket to the bed

do an all-night vigil outdoors

whip up a batch of blueberry muffins

discover the backstory of an object

feel your breath fill your lungs

decide to ask a question

wait for a butterfly to fly by

dance in a public fountain

vacuum the coils on the refrigerator

compile a book of unique recipes from
friends, family, and neighbors

try something new

discover how to train a bonsai tree

climb a hill

save electricity by unplugging all unused appliances

train for a marathon

begin a jigsaw puzzle

trace a hand turkey

dye your hair a crazy color

thank the cashier

bake a cake for no special reason

test the smoke and CO detectors

make a playlist of all your friends' favorite songs that you love

look at something out of context

write your autobiography

learn how to weave a basket

volunteer as a cuddler for premature infants

take up a hands-on hobby

use your best china

take care of a cactus

consider what could be instead of what is

sweep the floors

teach yourself a new skill

throw out crappy socks and underwear

stop and look at the view from a new window

tell a good story

go to the woods

spend the early morning commute observing

study a field guide for your region

sit on a lawn chair under a sprinkler

hide a coin in a busy public place you pass often

share your blessings

sneak a fast-food meal and hide the evidence

look at the backgrounds of photos

smell the aromas wafting through the air

adopt a good habit

look for a genuine arrowhead

sharpen the blunt crayons

teach someone to read or write

see what else an author has written

send a card for no obvious reason

see things as unfolding in their own time

seek out a view of late-afternoon slanting
    light

run in place

look for flower buds or new grass

replace a broken tile

organize a bookshelf, drawer, or closet

search for a mirage

renew your library card

make a Velcro target for sponge ball
    games

remove a dent

take a walking tour

reflect on all that is good in your life

rig a cat-feeding device

redecorate a corner of your home

create a word search puzzle

rearrange the books on a bookshelf in
    alphabetical order

listen to your inner voice and follow it

read to a kid

make a unique milkshake

remember the coupons

build a bat house

read an entry in a print encyclopedia

prep the garden

put things back where you found them

write a thank-you note

watch a woodpecker at work

do something your friends would
    describe as utterly unlike you

build a woodland den

pore over a favorite catalog

plan an adventure

pluck a hair and study it

create a recipe with your five favorite
foods

write a compliment to your neighbor and
leave it in the mailbox

go on an evening exploration, like a drive
in the country or a hike along a beach

do the yoga tree pose

paint the front door a bright color

prepare for an exam

reorganize the items on a shelf

open your eyes a little wider

practice for an athletic event

notice your spine as it leans against the
chair

play the dictionary game

notice something that is blossoming,
literally or figuratively

read all the Ellery Queen mysteries

notice a beautiful sky

perform a lucky ritual

nap in a tree

offer to dog-sit or dog-walk for a friend

meditate on a beautiful painting

offer a cold drink to a worker

massage your back with a tennis or
lacrosse ball

mend a fence

map the boring features of your
commute

read a writing style and usage manual

clean out your shoe collection

meditate in a Zen garden

master a classic sauce, such as
béarnaise

make and freeze homemade
dinners

look up, then look farther up

listen for bird language

put something attention-getting by the entrance to your home

light a candle at church

let a child do your hair

imitate a birdcall

get a tattoo removed

try different yoga styles

feel the wind in your hair

help someone assemble the ingredients for a recipe

learn about a different culture

have an art night with friends

jump rope

hang out at a bookstore

jump into a big pile of leaves

notice how it feels to go back and forth between sun and shade

jot down ideas for new beginnings

give away everything you have not worn in three years

join the library's summer book club

start a worm farm

plan a whole new look for yourself

donate your time to help a person or group

keep a wine journal

design a unique house

join an explorers club

get up and do something spontaneous

invite a friend over for chatting and snacks

remove a grass stain by using diluted white vinegar

indulge in a moment of silence before the first sip or bite

create a wish list of all the things you want to do or learn

identify the antecedent of a pronoun

get out of a stuffy room

read about the Enneagram

identify a big dream that will require your particular talents

finish up or dump that bottle of shampoo or that bar of soap

hit the bull's-eye on a dartboard

find new plants

spend time alone in the woods, just thinking

feed a hummingbird

examine the edges of a window

grow a fruit tree from seed

check the mousetrap

go outside and pay attention to one act of nature

dust the furniture

give your house the white-glove test

learn to whistle with your fingers

change the wreath on the front door

do a yucky chore and be glad it's done

give the cat a nighttime treat

drive around in a city

get some fresh air

dig out a piece of lawn and put in a
  garden

get ready for a trip

develop your own barbecue sauce recipe

unsubscribe from a mailing list

make a three-minute egg

hang up a bird feeder

get in synchronized step with someone

take a walk in the zoo

focus on each hair as you shave

practice concentrating by studying a rock
  for five minutes

plant a mini-garden in a glass jar

download a money management app and
  use it

paint a watercolor on the bedroom
  window

whittle a child's toy

go for a nature walk

compose a bouquet

follow the neighborhood cat

commit to a project

fold a paper airplane

carry a book with you

find something orange

have a winter barbecue

ask someone about their favorite smell

find a way to reuse something you were
originally going to throw away

explore a new area by bike

camp out in a state park

exercise at home

be a mentor

examine your cooking appliances
and get rid of ones you rarely or
never use

balance a book on your head for a half
hour

examine the veins of a fallen leaf

assemble a disaster kit or list

enjoy a good yawn

appreciate the consoling power of trees and clouds

eat the last piece of cake

write to a prisoner

figure out what work you'd like to have completed six months from now

consider five ways money can't buy joy

drop a dollar on the street and imagine who will find it and how they'll feel

winterize the car

drive a hard bargain

make a swear box

draw the ripples you see in a slow-moving brook

notice the world outside your window

draw something goofy in the margins of a notebook

look around for something yellow if you're feeling irritated or annoyed

draw an interminable staircase

weave a flower necklace

downsize your handbag

wave to people in other cars

donate books to a children's hospital

create a whiteboard for checking off chores

watch the world go by from a sidewalk café

learn how to wash windows correctly

try a sport that you are sure you would be terrible at

make your signature dish

eat at a groceraunt, a restaurant in a grocery store

wave at a passing train

donate a basketball to a local youth recreation center

water the grass

try office yoga at your desk

look for things to be happy about as you ride in a car

do things on your own

watch rain patter against the windshield

do nothing at all for at least 15 minutes

watch an aquarium or fishbowl

do an optional assignment

wash all the brushes and combs

dispose of old batteries properly

wash the car

discover something beautiful in an old familiar place

warm your feet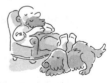

design the costumes for a Broadway musical

go to the same spot every day, noting the differences

come up with your own slang term

walk with a toddler

delight in a sunset

make a sundial for the backyard

walk up and down the stairs for
    10 minutes

decorate with books

declare a snow day and stay in bed

walk to town

dress up for a dress-down occasion

walk through a forest, observing wildlife

learn to dance the Charleston

walk on a rope

start a brand-new book

dance on a table

take out a paper map and find your way
    to a destination

cut your bangs

go for a walk at dawn

cut out a pattern

visit the historical society

sketch the bathroom of your dreams

visit an aquarium

create art with a kid

vacuum under a rug

craft a balsa-wood airplane

unload the dishwasher

count your blessings and round up

turn the Christmas lights on

pick a word at random in the dictionary
and use it in a sentence

make an outdoor obstacle course for a
pet or child

ask a rhetorical question

turn over the earth in the garden

cook with a friend

turn down the bedspread and prop up
the pillows

cook dinner for someone

turn a routine into a ritual

construct a card tower

try an extreme sport

combine an errand with something fun

transform your bedroom into a romantic haven

clear your cupboards of all the utensils and appliances you don't use

make a summer reading list

clear the driveway to play hoops

take a two-mile walk after lunch

clear out the old

touch your toes

chronicle your commute

time a traffic light

change what isn't working

tie a fishing fly

change a car's air filter

challenge yourself to find something lovely

create a well-stocked tool kit

celebrate the everyday

plan your funeral with no budget
restrictions

celebrate a self-invented holiday

listen to what other people want without
reacting, objecting, arguing, fighting,
or resisting

join a walking group

create an outdoor room for sleeping in
the summer

choose an unusual word to repeat
over and over until it sounds
ridiculous

teach your animal to do a trick

catch up on journaling

talk yourself into something

care for a neglected garden

take yourself on a playdate

make a move on your crush

look at water droplets traveling across your car window

call a friend

take off right now for a spur-of-the-moment adventure

build an elaborate construction out of Popsicle sticks

take note of all the interesting things you see, hear, smell, taste, and feel

brush your pet's teeth

take in whatever is unfolding in front of you

browse a brick-and-mortar store

write a thank-you letter to someone who influenced you

bring in logs from the woodpile

make a suggestion to the mayor

bring a blanket for a lunchtime picnic

watch a tired dog curl up and go to sleep

learn to whistle

do something you were never allowed to
do when you were young

play a word game

make one of the phone calls you dread
making 📱

build a stone wall on your property

become expert at croquet

take down the Christmas tree

learn a new Frisbee move

survey the horizon

be an active listener

surround yourself with beauty

be alert for curious and
unexpected smells

surprise someone

attempt to cut your own hair

put a tissue pack and lip balm in every
winter coat

open a thesaurus at random and learn
something

go on a walkabout

close your eyes, point to a place on a map, then go there

do the legs-up-the-wall yoga pose

check out what other shoppers have in their carts

submit a suggestion in a suggestion box

place each item in its proper place when unpacking groceries

stroll through a greenhouse

ask your mother or father the question you always wanted to ask

stretch your legs

arrange to have a professional organizer visit your home

stop thinking about whether you're doing it right

allow the character of a place to sink in slowly

stop the conversations that get replayed endlessly in your mind allow a simple, childlike wonder to overtake you

stop at a tag sale

admire a garden

steam your face over a pot of hot water

act on a great idea

make a sock monkey

re-grout tiles in the shower

stay up all night

create your own spaghetti sauce and personalize the jar

start keeping a record of your moods

picture your favorite scene

have a walking meeting rather than a sit-down meeting in an office or restaurant

record your dreams

find a way to reduce your negative impact on the environment

list things you like about yourself

stare into a fire and be mesmerized by the flames

look for old birds' nests, empty beehives, and vacant cocoons

stand on tiptoes

sort your books by subject

dance through the house

create storage for vital documents and let your family know

work because you want to

sponsor a kids' sports team

take pleasure in waiting

choose an absolute favorite work or exhibit in a museum or gallery

read a thesaurus page

pick up your walking pace

clean out your daypack

invent a silly walk

eat a thoughtfully prepared vegan meal

create your ultimate to-do list, one that helps you chart your path

split a banana split

make eating a pure focus activity

spend 20 minutes drinking a glass of water, noting everything about the activity

coax latent ideas to the forefront of your consciousness

stand in front of a piece of art that you think is boring and try to make it interesting

sort through holiday decorations and keep only the things you actually display

unclog a toilet or drain

sort the lingerie drawer

dress a scarecrow well

make a social call

find tasks to do at volunteer events

take a train to the end of the line, just to observe the people and scenery

recycle old textbooks

sit down and relax

make endless lists of things that are on your mind

sunbathe on the fire escape

dig through a rummage sale

find the suitcase key

review your lists

feel the way your cat settles into your lap

pause on the doorstep to sniff the air

sing a lullaby

tuck someone in

shop in a consignment store

learn how to wallpaper

shave a carrot

explore local landmarks

share an aha moment

bike through a city

sew on a button that's been missing

note which shoe you put on first

set the table

do vigorous aerobics for an hour

create a line of dominoes, then knock it down

move around your home décor rather than buying new objects

set aside a grudge

figure out what each person in a crowd of people has in common

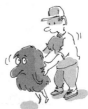

set an agenda

serenade your beloved

look for the unusual

practice self-control

start a tropical fish tank

work on your service game

plan a weekend of doing something
  you usually tell yourself you're too
  unadventurous for

try to spot a whale or shark

make a snow maze

take off your watch

keep a survival journal during hard times

finish a reading or assignment list

design a tablecloth

find an uplifting quotation or passage

find some Zen in the preparation of
  dinner

draw a series of things

decorate a white T-shirt

do jobs for the elderly

send the family off on a weekend trip

cut firewood

go to the movies solo

practice listening

send flowers to the one you love

archive your old work projects

garnish your next meal

send an appreciation card

design sneakers

select a paint color for a currently white or neutral room

do twice the number of sit-ups you think you can

get rid of things you don't use anymore

doodle

see the beauty in the water coming from the tap

unravel an unloved sweater and wind the yarn for a new project

see if you can pick the fastest lane or line

grow bamboo

see how far you can throw a paper airplane

count cricket chirps

sculpt a block of ice

follow marked trails

savor a long day

look at treetops out the window

run your fingers over smooth wood,
    stone, and other surfaces

return a smile

make a snow angel in the grass

make seven-layer dip

run through a field

name five things in a room and
    remember how they got there

run outside and say goodnight to the day

color-code books on your bookshelf

run a bath

turn off an unneeded light

paint recipe cards with watercolors as
    gifts

restore an antique frame

create a star system for recipes you have
tried in cookbooks

reorganize your closet

research a summer internship

rent a bicycle

write a review of a TV show you love

memorize where you parked the car

use flashcards on Varsity Tutors'
apps 📱

learn to use chopsticks properly

remember to turn out the
closet light

do a wheelie

put on your thinking cap

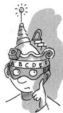

change the way your shoes
are laced

learn the North Star method
of navigation

help a stranger

explore the woods

catch a spelling error

categorize a collection

remember and plan for a birthday

audition for a play

refashion a T-shirt

donate something for an auction

rediscover a forgotten item of clothing in
your closet

connect with someone new

recall a lovely detail from your day

go birding

rearrange the furniture

walk the dog on a new route

convert waste materials or used products
into new materials or products

take a train by yourself to someplace you
have never been

amble in an unplanned or aimless way
with complete openness to the
unknown

make an intention to practice loving-
kindness and compassion

consider alternatives

read your electric meter

ice a cake

read something on the subway

send birthday cards to all your friends

read an entire book in a week

practice better handwriting or create
your own calligraphy style

act as if you know how to do something
that you actually don't know how to do

paint a watercolor at dawn

learn proper grammar

notice the veining in a slab of marble

create a theme park in your own
backyard

enjoy doing nothing

put down in words what you really want

go for doughnuts at the bakery

riff on a topic

read the first page of every book you own

identify what makes a vacation great,
then plan to do it

listen to what other patrons say to one
another or what the staff says to
them

chronicle history in a journal

read books on retirement options

gargle

offer to help without waiting for
someone to ask

reschedule an appointment for a more
convenient time

rake the carpet

babysit for someone who needs a break

have a theme for the day

make paper plate Frisbees

find a very dark place to look at the stars
in silent solitude

assemble ingredients to make a meal

make a snack

wash out the bathing suits

raise your cultural literacy

rub soap on drawer edges so they will not stick

put one foot in front of the other, over and over

sort, purge, assign a home to, and containerize

put an ice cube on your hand and watch it melt

notice everything around you that is not art

put all the mini things you have in a maxi jar

divest your life of the superfluous

pursue your artistic bent

deal with a middleman/middlewoman

pull out a board game and call it game night

sit under a tree and enjoy the fresh air

provide a frog or turtle with safe crossing

write a fan letter to your favorite writer

visit a working farm

watch a thunderstorm

talk to yourself

do something you haven't done in years

pretend you do not speak English

build a stone column

play a version of I Spy using colors

follow a wave or a ripple, start to finish

find your way with a map and compass

explore a parking lot

discover a tickle spot

complete a project

change your sleep schedule

plan what you'd like to go back to
    school for

propose a controversial idea

wait out a sudden downpour

preserve a flower

thaw the frozen meat or dessert

make a smoothie

learn efficient note-taking

practice Christmas carols

accomplish things while sitting on
a porch

pore over old files to spark an idea

jot a note on a cocktail napkin

put a stash of toys in the guest room

cross-dress for a day

go on a vision quest

reminisce

do the cat-cow yoga pose

learn something by watching the
goings-on around you

ponder today's successes and tomorrow's
prospects

collect pinecones

polish the furniture

invite a neighbor in for coffee

play What am I?

cook without a recipe

plan your dream for the night

meditate under the stars

create a terrarium

destroy photos that make you look terrible

use a new spice

remember your glasses

watch the wind blow through a tree's branches

pick someone's brain

try a new restaurant

use a jeweler's loupe or magnifying glass to closely examine something

make your partner's favorite snack or meal

do high-intensity interval training

figure out your priorities

open stuck windows

place your hands in namaste, the position of respect and gratitude

donate your old books

picnic in a country meadow

interrupt constancies and equilibriums in the interest of new possibilities

make a shrine on the top shelf of a bookcase

dive under a wave

color in a structured pattern, like a mandala

look for the positive

arrange the vegetables on your plate in concentric circles

pick the lint off clothes

power walk

people-watch at the diner

organize your shoes

peer into puddles

manage your investment portfolio

pause for reflection

train volunteers

imagine what another person is thinking

invite your waitress or waiter to sit and
visit with you for a few minutes

make a crooked part in your hair

enter the space of a painting

part with fashion mistakes

break down a task into subcomponents

pare down the keys you carry

check on the children

paint with water

take out the garbage

paint in the garden

donate the remains of a garage sale to
a thrift shop

take a swim

paint an acrylic design on a flower vase

mow the lawn in a pattern

take out a library book on how to do
    something new

try a new method to unwind

read a textbook

clean out your cabinets

go to a museum and pick your top
    10 favorite things

create the perfect comeback for the last
    argument you had

walk on a treadmill

make a ship in a bottle

treat yourself to room service

take an online IQ test

set up camp

put together an Erector set

put the toilet seat down

prepare a weekly menu

improve your spelling

get to work early

focus on your breathing

fix a zipper

design your wedding rings

count the waves

stick something under a wobbly table leg

pack your backpack for the entire day
and go

mow and edge the yard

pack for a trip

follow a curious impulse

observe what goes on in a food court or
coffee shop

note a bird's arrival, process, and
departure

look at things from someone else's
perspective

evaluate a problem

create a *temenos*, a sacred space for
mental work

surprise your partner with a candlelight dinner

observe how art changes depending on the distance you are from it

iron a button-down shirt

notice when you are happy

go tanning

notice things at dawn that get missed in the rush of the day

find the silver lining in the cloud

negotiate a difference of opinion

feel the warmth of your partner's hand

name three of Aesop's fables

listen very quietly in total darkness or in a very large room

memorize your lines for a play

register for pet therapy training

make a shell necklace

chant the vowels of any language you know, in any order

memorize a poem by Walt Whitman

landscape the yard

line all your clothes drawers with
    scented paper

pick fruit in an orchard

measure your biceps

appreciate a pause to do nothing

sound out a tune on a piano

accept the highway traffic at rush hour

make an orienteering course

capture creative ideas on the fly

ask a question you would not ordinarily
    ask

fold clothes like origami

master the art of single-tasking

perform the Jedi mind trick

make two casseroles and take one to
    a friend or neighbor

thread a needle with the thread you most
    often use

make someone smile

name a baby

throw a TGIF party

order colors from favorite to least
favorite

find a treasure on the street

calibrate the oven

make juice from fruit

rummage through a shelf of old books in
an antique store

make Christmas cards

bone up on an interesting subject

start a tradition of celebrating
half-birthdays

bake brownies

plan a vacation

pour cream into a cup of iced coffee
and enjoy the swirl

keep a seashell collection at the beach

pop corn

make a series of drawings of each and
every thing in your field of vision

organize kitchen cookware by size
and shape

take a survival course

aid and abet a good deed

design a stage set

catch someone's eye from across
the room

make as little sound as possible

stretch a sore muscle

create some friendly drama

look out a window and realize you
have no control over what
you will see

walk laps at the track

learn Latin equivalents for things you
say all the time

locate a focal point

rent an RV and go on a road trip

list the contents of every storage box in the garage on its side

greet a delivery person you've been waiting for to save them a few steps

list 100 good things that have happened in your life

detach from your thoughts by watching them

line up a new project

crochet an afghan

lie in a meadow, forget everything, and feel the sun on your skin

toss popcorn into the air and catch it in your mouth

lick the cake bowl and beaters

get lost in a library

let the dog out

realize what Facebook and Twitter really are

warm someone's cold hands

let go

make mud pies

leave funny messages on sugar packets
in restaurants

count backward

leave flowers on a coworker's desk

return favors

listen to water

get rid of things you've been
keeping "just in case"

join a softball league

volunteer at the local nursing home

make a seed ball and throw it where
you can watch the seeds grow

take the subway to a non-destination

organize a refrigerator filled with
everything you like

solve a word puzzle

choose a theme song for yourself

pretend to be asleep

play with your kids on Saturday

plant a tree

empty your pockets

list all the things you did well today

learn a tongue twister

get your ice skates sharpened

drive to the road's end

decide what you would do if you won
the lottery

cook a romantic meal

press the auto clean button on the oven

check the woodpile

attend a social event

root around in the back of your closet

learn what all the lights mean on your
dashboard

start the coffee maker

watch worms work

deliberate over a decision

leaf through a slim volume of verse

draw tree bark magnified 1,000 times

write a sonnet, a 14-line poem

collect bait at night for morning fishing

watch a snail slowly make its way to its
destination

consume M&M's by color groups

make a seed and pasta picture

watch dragonflies

do something you enjoy that your
partner or friends do not

transplant a cutting from a houseplant

build a snow penguin

tie your shoelaces a different way than
usual

learn to twirl, dip, and delay a Frisbee

talk about happy things

learn Japanese ink wash painting

do three types of exercise today

change the way you respond to your
thoughts

shine a pair of shoes

play kick the can

batten down the hatches

look for the oldest thing around you

stack rocks to form unique sculptures

lie down and melt into the floor

excuse a blunder

keep an illustrated journal

exercise your lungs with rhythmic breathing

look up how to tie four really handy knots 📱

jump as high as you can

drink straight from a coconut

observe something about everything in your field of vision

invite people over for a coffeehouse evening

frame something you painted

invite friends for a hike

land a skateboard trick

learn to crochet toys for your pet

desalinate the coffee machine

hug a pillow

introduce a dietary change

fly a homemade kite

install a clothesline

cleverly disguise electrical cords and
 cables

place a letter stamp upside down to
 signify love

study Greek to improve your knowledge
 of English

go on a silent, meditative hike

play an instrument

make a scratching post for the cat

send mental messages to someone

take a stress test

pit the cherries

do the worst task first

learn by copying

throw your hat in the ring

open a sketchbook and sketch the first
   thing you see

plan birthday and holiday shopping early

go to the gym

mail envelopes to fake addresses in
   different countries and see if they
   come back

close your eyes to savor an experience

discard all food that makes you feel
   clogged up, toxic, sluggish, or fat

check out what everyone is wearing

practice creative waiting

"lose" marbles in a public place knowing
   someone will find them

scratch an itch

practice using a fire extinguisher

imagine your ideal lifestyle

plan for your golden years

find odd words in your dictionary

illustrate your favorite book

paint a wall an unusual color

have dinner as a family

notice the unfurling of a blossom

practice some basic carpentry skills

identify your mission in life

go for a walking meal, stopping for
    different courses along the way

record metaphor-free observations
    about your world

hop a fence

exercise your fingers

hold the door open for someone

do something especially odd for you

hold an indoor treasure hunt

look toward true north

hire someone to rake and clean up the
    leaves

send in warranty cards

make a schedule for sending birthday
    cards on time

inner-tube down snowy hills

hike a cool trail

forgive and forget

help the environment

ask yourself, "What am I really craving?"

illustrate a journal

look at the wild meadow beyond

have breakfast in bed

memorize phone numbers

greet the letter carrier

spin wool

have a staring contest with someone

do woodworking

find a treasure in the attic

spend five minutes looking to the left,
    then five minutes looking to the
    right, and write about the differences

go swimming

braise meat

go someplace cold

**turn your refrigerator door
  into an art gallery**

roll dice to make a decision

go see some live entertainment

mulch leaves

go over work materials in a park

overtip a waitress or waiter

brave the weather

go home and relax

segment a grapefruit

create a sport that is playable in your
  office or studio

help preserve a landmark

go downtown

fixate on a solution

go camping

make jam or preserves

provide a take-along meal for a friend
   going on a flight

dispense useless facts

make a scarecrow

make egg salad

get something fixed

rally around someone who needs a boost

read a table of contents

wash the towels

pick up trash off the streets
   and dispose of it properly

throw a surprise party

invent a secret code

think of what you would do if you had
   only three months to live, then do it

eat a square of chocolate mindfully

teach a dog a new trick

create your own wrapping paper

sit in silence for 15 minutes

bake a loaf of bread

set a timer for 30 minutes and do not
  check it

read the safety instructions card

share your happiness with someone else

plan the upcoming week

perfect your tennis serve

participate in your neighborhood watch

organize a voter registration drive

name your rock band

make sure your will is in order and up
  to date

leave a used book where someone will
  discover it

hang a tire swing

make plans with two of your coworkers

give yourself the free time you need to
  explore

fill out the "How was the service?" card

do an oral history project

discover the surprise waiting in your workday

decide to start a new habit first thing in the morning

dance in the street

make a sand painting and then layer the extra sand by color in a sealable jar

compile a list of all the airports you have landed in or left from

take a spelling quiz

climb a tree in a public place

make a ridiculous bet with a friend

seek spaces where you would create street art

share a quiet moment

adopt a tree and get to know it

get really good meat from the butcher

light a scented candle and close your eyes

get from A to B using a paper map

sunbathe

get a stain out

organize your underwear drawer

cook a meal mindfully

find the receipt you need for a return,
    repair, or replacement

massage your feet and hands with
    lotion

mow the lawn and feel the vibration of
    the mower

create some semblance of order

gaze at a candle flame as meditation

watch a video on how to twirl and toss
    a baton 📱

gather the documents you need to
    prepare your taxes

do a stream-of-consciousness exercise

gain the knack of reading upside down

nibble carrots or celery sticks

frolic in leaves

frame a certificate

envision your retirement

follow your bliss

acknowledge good things
    about your partner

create a space to do yoga

practice Zenlike concentration

learn how to use a caulk gun

ask how someone is and actually wait for
    the answer

watch the surf for an hour

build muscles

make a salad

juggle rolled-up socks

chase dragonflies and fireflies

try a new recipe

dabble with felt-tip pens

listen to ambient noise

make your own soap

speak an affirmation aloud to your
    reflection in a mirror

figure out where the psoas muscles are

induce a trance state

fold and put away your clothes

donate winter coats

incorporate art into your journal

flip through a book, choose a phrase, and
decide what it means to you

remove nail polish

fix up an old car

plan a visit to a college friend

finish an entire puzzle book

clear paths in a park

find things to scratch your back against

park your car somewhere and just sit

look for the oldest exhibit item in a
museum

draw a piece of toast

find inspiration from something nearby

rewrite the copy on the back of a
cereal box

start a recycling project

ask directions, even if you're not lost

plan a trip

practice music scales

fix something

keep a record of gifts given to avoid giving the same thing again

post a sign warning against cell phone use in cars

design a sarong

throw open the shutters, curtains, or windows

make a rubber band ball

precook part of a meal

work on your novel

make recipe cards

try to remember your lock combination

declutter for 15 minutes

page through an encyclopedia volume, reading whatever catches your eye finish a project early

beat up your pillow

find an old toy or game you forgot about

install a faucet aerator

enjoy the sunshine

write a song for somebody

draw a self-caricature or self-portrait

watch a rainbow till it disappears

decorate a tablecloth or place mats

do something you don't usually have
time for

file your nails

build a shoebox house or diorama

establish an emergency fund

prioritize the day's tasks

establish a calming routine that you can
use if you feel yourself getting angry

dice onions

go to the beach

donate proceeds from a yard sale to a charitable organization

engage in manual labor

come up with neat things to use as bookmarks

embroider a jock for a jock

create mnemonics to remember your passwords

discover or declare something new about yourself

pick something up with your toes

create a spa day

read roadside markers

eavesdrop on nature without disturbing its daily routine

broach a sensitive subject with sensitivity

make a reverse layup in basketball

slice fruit or vegetables

take a solo road trip

blow bubbles

have a snowball fight

organize cosmetics

be kind to an animal

find a stranger to smile at

accessorize your outfit

get rid of the stuff you do not need

bird-watch

traverse a hay or corn maze

soften your facial muscles

eat under a tree

say grace

eat only one color for a meal

jump in a mud puddle

keep a notebook of ongoing lists of
people, places, and things that
interest you

file children's keepsakes

eat an all-dessert dinner

learn dining etiquette

deconstruct a scene as you imagine
a historian would

bring coffee to someone in bed

put a sketchbook in your purse or
backpack

create a 15-minute silent retreat

blaze a trail

create exotic life stories for people who
walk by

dwell in stillness

send a handwritten thank-you note

look at the western sky in midevening

watch what's cooking in the oven

dust off an old musical instrument

make s'mores

drop your thoughts into a journal

host a poker night, using M&M's as
poker chips

make a restaurant reservation

eat your favorite comfort food for dinner

drive with all the windows open

clean obsolete papers out of your files

make checklists

drink coffee and write poetry at a diner

get artsy-craftsy

do a taste test of bottled and tap water

watch raindrops race each other down
the window

dream up names for future kids

explore unfamiliar parts of your town

draw your pet while it's sleeping

read tea leaves

draw inspiration from photographs

solve a Rubik's Cube

draw in the dark

pull the curtains open

doze in a chair in front of the fireplace

include back exercises in an abdominal workout

donate toys to a day care center or children's hospital

size up the competition

donate your clutter to charity

assign colors to the days of the week

begin a journal of a baby's first year

weed between the patio rocks

do what is possible

regard each footstep as a unique event

do tasks and get them out of the way

camp out in your car

pick an event from your day and imagine describing it to an alien

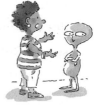

explore rock pools

tolerate silence

pick a topic and study it in depth

create a snow sculpture

take inventory of everything you see in
 a waiting room

make art out of recycled items

ask a question, then be silent while it is
 answered

do a standing forward bend

use a travel journal

change the way you feel by changing the
 way you act

train a pet

remember to set the alarm

throw away old sponges

put on the kettle

tell someone your (age-appropriate!)
 fantasies

look up the names of five birds indigenous
 to your area 📱

take something upstairs

help a neighbor

study the teachings of the Buddha

explore the universe through a telescope

stop to notice an instance of natural beauty

catch a possibility as it passes

stare at your toes or fingers and note the similarities and differences between them

tell someone a story

take care of the little things before taking care of the big things

spend a lunch hour in a beautifully planted atrium

practice a three-point basketball shot

play in the snow

pay attention to what you pay attention to

pack a surprise in a lunch or snack bag

observe a yoga, Pilates, or exercise class you might like to take

make up a song about your family

hunt for numbers

plan a themed dinner

have your tires rotated

go through your wardrobe and donate
the things you will never wear again

give a lottery ticket to a stranger

get someone to throw a Frisbee with you

focus on your sense of touch

fill the sugar canister

learn how to tie scarves cleverly

make potpourri

fill a rumbly tummy

take a solo expedition to explore
something rare or unusual

experiment with new ideas in how you
dress

allow yourself to dream

use your finger to spell out a message on
a friend's back

donate an unused swing set to a day care
center

do your shopping at a farmers market

clean up the workbench

buy a surprise book for someone

build something with a kid

ask questions to gain more insight

read a spooky book while a storm is
    brewing

ask for what you want

draw on the night sky with a sparkler

arrange a potluck party

alternate between reading a short story
    and an essay

dress up the dog

admire someone's teeth

add a waypoint to the map

do somersaults down a grassy hill

challenge someone to a race

do the Pilates tabletop exercise

gather wood to start a fire

accomplish one thing really well

select a color or shape and look for it
everywhere

paint a bland wooden chair a bright color

line the walkway to your house with
luminaria

notice the tiny details of drawings

play old maid

go for a walk without direction

explore someplace new

get back to people right away

have a water gun fight

make a plot for a garden

paint snow using a spray bottle filled
with water and food coloring

create a silk flower arrangement

smell for changes in the weather

go grocery shopping

swap reading lists with friends

do everything in slow motion

row a boat

refresh the dried spices

dissect a chicken nugget

recycle wrapping paper

listen to the wind

collect factoids

give yourself a physical challenge

join a social organization that serves the community

discover new insights

plant an organic garden

dine by candlelight

diagram a sentence

collect seedpods from trees and grow them in pots

detox after a large meal

catch snatches of sleep in the passenger's seat

note the most inexplicable and unlikely object you can see

write or draw your current feelings

look for the newest thing around you

have a silent contest with someone

complete four tiny tasks

find a story with a happy ending and
    read it

label things

decorate your bike or skateboard

give yourself a pedicure

decorate paper bags for lunches

find the quiet center within yourself

make a pledge to public radio

feel yourself connected to the center of
    the earth via gravity

declutter your cubicle or office

dry summer flowers for winter bouquets

go to sleep early

play shadow charades

dance with your child

say hi to a stranger

dance to the beat of a different drummer

knit

dance a jig

reactivate your gym membership

cut up six-pack rings before disposing to help save marine life

laugh at yourself

cut that errant toenail

snack on high-protein foods

cut a balloon free from a car sales lot

make double, freeze half

cultivate your garden

boil an egg

choose something to do only while doing your laundry and call it "the laundry project"

pilfer a cookie

crash a party

bounce Silly Putty or a Super Ball

crack open a new book

scout things to draw

cozy up to your partner

satisfy your sweet tooth with fruit

count how many people are in line

negotiate for something you want

write a six-word memoir

eat all your popcorn before the movie
   starts, then get more

watch a quiet snowfall

crawl back under the covers

create a palindrome

practice mindful sitting

make a Play-Doh sculpture

create a silhouette portrait

compose riddles with elegant solutions

take a Slinky for a walk

imitate everyday sounds

build a sandcastle

experiment in the kitchen

visit a pet store with tropical fish

learn to speed-read

talk to your pet

do a stage spin

pretend you are on a desert island

play a tune on water glasses

break one of your own rules

organize the medicine cabinet

look at the stars through a telescope

make the perfect grilled cheese sandwich

eat potato chips one by one, listening to
the crunch

follow a star till you get home

donate blood

study with someone

walk in the forest, finding your way with
natural markers

explore a new park

provision a root cellar

start a new painting

build a safety shelter

read Aristotle or Plato

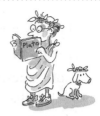

plan a safari of mystical creatures

fine-tune an idea

eat in a crowded restaurant or cafeteria without company—human or electronic

chase a butterfly

design a sales brochure

take five deep breaths

discover a star to wish upon

discuss an interesting topic

make a plan to hike the Appalachian, Continental Divide, or Pacific Crest trails

cash in your piggy bank or coin jar

complete a painting

paint watercolor greeting cards

change your routine

create a Pinterest board 📱

cook something in the oven that you
usually microwave

assess how point of view shapes the
content and style of an article

cook for the church supper

get certified in first aid

consult a fortune-teller

observe all the details of your hands

put a sketch pad next to the bed

find somewhere to be alone

go on a secret mission

convince everyone to play charades

find your way home

open a new container of something

uncap the pen and start writing

close your eyes to hear the wind rustle
the trees

watch butterflies play tag

check out the people at a public event—
who looks familiar and why?

decide which ancient or antique book
you'd like to have

consider what thing in your environment
will outlast everything else in the
scene

drag out an old washtub, sit under a tree,
and tip a hose in

confide in a diary

paper a small wall with art posters

concoct a dream in which you are an
archaeologist digging for artifacts

glimpse moments of lives unfolding
through windows

concentrate on an indoor hobby

strip furniture

compliment a friend

devise a method to stop biting your nails

communicate with an animal

rethink a long-held opinion

make a place in the garden for contemplation

identify one thing you have taken for granted your entire life

commit to spending at least an hour a week investing in your artistic growth

eat your next meal in silence, truly savoring and appreciating the food

create a secret handshake

split firewood

rehearse for a play or memorize a soliloquy

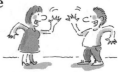

watch the sun move across the sky for at least 10 minutes

walk slowly enough to smell the flowers

try a new idea

run

make your own pickles

bat around an idea

figure out what your pain is trying to tell you

lower the blinds

combine different cereals in one bowl

watch pizza being made

collect your childhood drawings

get rid of the negativity of the day

collect and arrange seashells, pebbles, autumn leaves, or dried weeds

stand up straighter

collapse in bed and cuddle

finger-paint

collaborate on a puzzle

order takeout

coin a word or phrase for something that bothers you

cultivate ambidexterity

clip your fingernails

breathe the wild air

imagine what job you'd moonlight for fun and profit

clean and lubricate your bicycle

reclaim underused spaces for natural habitats

clean all the baseboards

hug someone

make a pilgrimage

coax elusive memories to return

take a hike in the rain

rake an elderly person's leaves

choreograph a dance

collect odd facts

chat with a docent

enjoy what you are reading for the beauty of the language

look for the good in this moment

watch someone being creative

check your arithmetic

choose the longest checkout line, then breathe slowly, accepting your impatience

exercise a whole different set of muscles

cheer up a dreary desk with flowers or something colorful

scrub your face

break your big goals into smaller steps

check to see if the mail has arrived

do leg lifts

have a rotten day party

place flowers on an unattended gravestone

find a sport you enjoy

design doghouses and cat perches

check for monsters under the bed

remember all the words to your favorite song

choose to get wet in the rain

imagine someone playing a very long
    note on a violin

chat up the checkout person

plant rogue bulbs and wildflowers

chase the cat so you both get exercise

start becoming the change you want to
    see in the world

buy a new doormat

wear socks that don't match

celebrate an accomplishment

make plans you can look forward to

defend yourself

get rolfed

make a piece of art inspired by your
    favorite artist

give to the needy

catch an insect inside the house,
    then release it outside

unclutter your most cluttered room

catalog a library

play mah-jongg

create a rotating six-year tax file

do extra homework

carve out time for your dreams

see something you are not actually
looking at

carve a jack-o'-lantern for Halloween

carry bags of groceries for someone

capture the day's best moments in
writing

walk or run up a hill, then run down
really fast, and repeat

bury your nose in flowers

skip down the middle of the street

bundle up for a hike

create autumn leaf art

brush the cat

complete a crossword puzzle without
looking at the answers

get on a plane to see someone

go to sleep

race up or down the stairs

learn to slam-dunk

update your travel toiletries kit

do a special project that you have been
putting off

draw Pokémon

listen to the shower water as it falls

write your will

read a short novel in a long day

volunteer as part of a community service
program

ask yourself, "What would a child see
here?"

clean under your bed

use your label maker

change the voice in your head to a more
positive one

try loving what you have

come up with five positive thoughts for every negative one

email a teenager something you wish you had known as a teen

make a personal save-the-planet list

study a photograph

pick up the newspaper from the driveway

spend time with a funny person

invent a sandwich

sneak a Popsicle before dinner

eat a sandwich on the steps of a museum

try to identify the spices in a hot dish

create your own version of a recipe

sharpen the tools

write down three things that made you happy today

send a pebble skipping across a pond

walk a shoreline

seek out wild paths

treat yourself to breakfast out

seek awe in the sky, a sunrise, or a storm rolling in

take an interest in others' lives

set up an indoor obstacle course

rig a zip line

put the ski rack on the car

remember the umbrella

prepare a treasure hunt for a birthday party

read the index of a book

improve your signature

put the things you use most often in the easiest-to-find places

get to know your teachers

try something new on your toast

focus on how you can make a difference

pull a weed and get all the roots with it

fix a spot on the wall with acrylic paint

prepare for tomorrow

design a wedding dress or suit

practice for the school play or concert

make a personal map, maybe of the places the cat enjoys in your home

play the teacups

take a shower

perform a task in silence

look at the eye color of everyone in your vicinity

offer to run an errand for someone

count the stars until you lose count

offer a toast at dinner

create a rock garden

mend a quarrel

write a sitcom based on your life

master a yo-yo trick

watch a pickup game of basketball at the neighborhood park

look up words in a physical dictionary

do something generous and keep it a secret

get the sprinkler going

light a fire in the hearth

build a rock wall

imitate a funny scene from a movie

find the point of perspective in
a painting

help someone work on a project

feel the sun and breeze on your body

have an intimate talk with a parent

hang out with your kid

plan a visit to your hometown

give away five things you do not need

get an unpleasant thing over with

finish the unfinished

use a grill to make dessert

feed a stranger's expired parking meter

examine the medicine cabinet items'
expiration dates

paint a stormy scene

perfect a velouté sauce

notice the texture of the food
   you eat

empty the wastebaskets

go for a walk at lunchtime

dust the top of the refrigerator

drive around with the windows down
   on a late summer night

make a wading pool in the sand

develop your spiritual practice

learn how to throw a curveball

develop some general but meaningful
   questions to ask at meetings

compose a perfect haiku

stay mentally present for your workout

carry a paperback book to read
   throughout the day

camp out under the dining
   room table

be a tourist in your own town

balance a stack of stones or pebbles

assemble a toy

get up early enough to join the regulars for breakfast at the local coffee shop

appreciate the space between appointments on your calendar

build on ideas to make better ideas

invent a stage name

create an alias

note the things around you that deserve a compliment

make an inventory of every item you own in a single category

make coleslaw

ask a person to tell you a story from their youth

divide your to-do list into vital, necessary, and trivial

brown-bag it and take a walk

pan for gold or minerals

bring your attention to your breath while
waiting in line

do a little favor for someone

bring someone a box of chocolates for
no reason at all

repaint a door

watch stars twinkle

break out into a run

pitch an indoor camp

make a perfect over-easy egg

lie down and roll over

put a rug down for bare feet

plan a road trip with a child

compose yourself over coffee

do the unexpected

have a reverse dinner, dessert first

develop the left side of your brain by
playing chess

compose poems between stoplights

create a reading nook

crack an egg perfectly

find a shortcut

dig until you find buried treasure

bow to the morning sun

get on the floor and stretch

bounce a basketball

approach the next task with reverence

spot a hidden flower

speak like Yoda

blow the down off dandelion heads

stand on a small massage ball to unlock
your tense foot muscles

bike to the beach or market

ford a river

start a new mission

dedicate an hour to watch the sunrise at
dawn

accept the weather without looking at
a forecast

catch thoughts in a notebook

carve an eraser to make an ink stamp

design a ring

float your hands through tall milkweeds
or corn stalks

work on your magnum opus

exercise outside

try to reconcile two enemies

learn to skateboard

make a nest for humans on the living
room floor using pillows and blankets

make a self-portrait in the snow

take a sensory walk, during which you
focus only on smell

choose a new recipe for dinner from a
cookbook

do a face mask

get something new and give something
away

find an old scrapbook

offer suggestions for town improvements

draw a piece of furniture as you are
looking down on it

clip coupons

begin a new book with no obligation to
finish it

write a short story outdoors, using your
surroundings as inspiration

befriend a reference librarian

personalize your handbag

swap goods and services

become aware of personal strengths you
did not know you had

beautify your handwriting

make, modify, repair, or reuse what you
already have

beat a new path

leave a friendly surprise in the mailbox
for the letter carrier

bask in the glow of a roaring fire

cross a line you haven't crossed before

balance on one foot

find everything you need in the cupboard
for a new recipe

attune yourself to birdsong

play pub trivia

take your sketchbook
out for dinner

attack a canvas with fearlessness

housebreak or house-train a pet

make a pending box for loose papers in
your home or office

try indoor rock climbing

go to see a stone quarry

tune up your bicycle

assign a name to your state of mind

repay a kindness

choose a project from an arts and crafts
website 📱

drive some exciting roadways through
 towns and areas you have not seen

send postcards

smell your partner's hair or your pet's fur

create a raised-bed garden

pamper yourself

re-create a special date or occasion

ask about someone's day and listen to the
 nuance of the answer

disambiguate the meaning of a word you
 use often

swab the decks

approach a person with curiosity

pet an animal

name two things you can hear in
 the room

appreciate your essential nothingness

find two good reasons to do something

appreciate an artful display

hang upside down

apply for a passport

read philosophy

listen to the sound of a leaf falling
through tree limbs

dry someone's wet shoes

arrange pillows

join a singing group

draw faces on the undersides of
your toes

create an oasis of calm in your day

play air guitar

make a paperweight

reseed bare patches of lawn

test a multistep skincare routine

rediscover your muse

volunteer at the library

recycle everyday stuff into artwork

take the stairs

shovel snow

solve a riddle

bleach your whites

pretend to be an alien fresh off the
spaceship

seek an oddball, out-of-the-way place to
eat in an obscure neighborhood

play with somebody else's stuff

plant a seed in a paper cup

look through the wrong end of
a telescope

hide the remote control

identify a risk you'd like to take but are
afraid to

remember a good joke

learn to say hello in a new language

pump iron

get your hair cut

refurbish a flea market find

drive to the ocean at sunrise

race a bike

decide what you would do if you were invisible for a day

cook a perfect omelet

become active in volunteer work

clean your kitchen with all-natural ingredients

mend a pair of beloved jeans

dig the wax out of a candlestick holder

cleanse, tone, and moisturize your face

read a provocative article in a business journal

plan the perfect ski trip

paint by number

sight or cite at least one thing that makes you happy

take a road trip making only left turns

mark all your junk mail "return to sender"

meet a deadline

check the list twice

identify one good thing about your job

attend a service of another religion

look for coins in the couch

note what you'd wish you'd done more of
    if tomorrow were your last day
    on earth

embroider a hand towel

answer a letter

admire the extraordinary light of the sun

label containers and boxes in the closet

create a private sanctuary

keep the scorebook or scorecard

learn how to swim

watch the spaces between people

try a new hairstyle

write backward

make your own granola

go singing and puddle-jumping in the
    rain

figure out what is the farthest thing you can see clearly from where you are

increase your vocabulary with five new words

allow your eyes to relax and focus on nothing

master parallel parking

write a science fiction novel

look up and sketch Zentangle tiles 📱

watch a patch of melting snow

deliver on a promise

do a self-check-in and figure out what makes you want to scroll

realize how lucky you are

have a really honest conversation

read someone's mind

make a one-pot meal

find a secret place to write

look outside

take a multivitamin

make lemon curd

get homework done before you leave school

allow time for mind play, like a crossword or jigsaw puzzle

put plants in the bathroom

identify cloud formations

air out the quilts

sit near a pond and watch the sunlight on the water

saunter

learn to shuffle and deal cards expertly

play croquet

do a simple activity just for the joy of doing it

change the car's spark plugs

get a close look at a bird while it is nesting

put on self-tanning lotion

adjust a handbag strap to the ideal length

learn the names of your letter carrier and UPS driver

add to someone's collection

volunteer to help a friend move

add an *o* to the end of a word to make more colorful, e.g., *dangerouso*

explore the unbeaten path

adapt a monastic practice of contentment

catch a leaf as it is falling from a tree

act ridiculously to cheer someone up

register to vote, or help someone clse to

cross-stitch

acknowledge a job well done

make three wishes

observe the lines of buildings

rub two sticks together and start a fire outside

conjure metaphors

invite someone to sleep over

make a bracelet from things found on
a nature walk

act yourself into a new way of thinking

reach toward a new aspiration

follow an online makeup tutorial

stash a love note where your partner will
find it

find the perfect thing to wear

read a comic book

skewer meat and vegetables to grill

make soup from scratch

get directions

cast with a fly rod

make Jell-O

scratch someone's back, literally or
figuratively

just breathe

create a private language

wrap presents

arrange store-bought flowers

visit someone who would love to
see you

make a new friend

waterproof your shoes

rework a piece of writing

make a list of 10 things you'd keep if you
got rid of everything else

arrange something fun to look forward to

shut your office door and take a nap

bring crystals and semiprecious stones
into your home

watch bird behavior

put a plant in the sunlight

barbecue under the moon

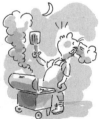

go on an overnight road trip
with no destination

put trash into trash receptacles

do the total opposite of what you had
planned

take detailed mental photographs of a moment

open a nearby window to let in sounds and smells

redesign an everyday product

power walk at the track

take a pottery class

observe thoughts as if they are passing clouds

close your eyes for 60 seconds, then open them to see what has changed

wander a museum wing

check out the old neighborhood

alternate two physical activities, such as yoga and walking

donate used bikes

re-caulk the bathtub

track shark sightings with Sharktivity

pre-steam fresh young vegetables

practice the camel yoga pose

get a bank employee to explain a CD until
   you understand it

donate free time

sit in a church during off hours

strum a ukulele

help out on a farm

stock up on provisions

admire things from afar

come up with rhyming epitaphs

save the life of an ant

oil a squeaky door

give extra kisses

use a walk among trees and flowers as
   aromatherapy

make potato prints

untangle a knot

fulfill an obligation

skim print newspaper headlines

skinny-dip

chronicle an exciting scene

get closure on something that has been troubling you

invent road trip games

speed walk

focus all your thoughts on your breathing

document your travels

make a motivation board

shampoo the dog

set a timer and accomplish something before it beeps

breakfast by candlelight on a dark morning

unkink a kinked cord

take boxing lessons

paint a still life

bank the fire in a woodstove or fireplace

notice the sensation of your hands when holding something

use international trailblazing symbols of grass, sticks, and rocks on your walk

go for a walk and find the quietest spot

jog with a pet or friend

record a podcast episode

contemplate rocks created four hundred million years ago

design shoes

hum a waltz

enter your name in a local sweepstakes

refill your pen

create a poster

stand like a mountain—feet apart, arms up in the air

experiment to find the best recipe

crush herbs with a mortar and pestle

start a neighborhood watch group

become invisible for a while

plan a perfect day in your head

throw darts at the pub

create a maintenance log for your home

watch lightning from a faraway thunderstorm

design a retreat for yourself

create freeform origami

tap out a message in Morse code

prune the trees

lay out your morning coffee's ingredients

use small seashells as vases for tiny flowers

neaten your cuticles

read a historical plaque

make a miniature version of something

campaign for a cause you believe in

listen to the ocean in a shell

follow that little dirt road, zigzagging off in search of adventure

repair your own eyeglasses

define the ingredients of a good life

add five items to the end of this book

learn Esperanto

dance and laugh with a kid

play among big trees and rocks

organize your vitamin and medicine cabinet

stroke a dog's ears

replace one unhealthy aspect of your life with a healthy one

unclench your teeth

look at the center of a very small object

illuminate a favorite painting

silence a squeaky floor

practice mental arithmetic

read ingredient labels

exfoliate

put new laces in your shoes and boots

canoe

draw something that looks realistic

unstick something that is stuck

have a really good photograph taken
of you

practice running backward

find a reminder system that works

do a sardine meditation in a crowded
situation ("we are all alike and in the
same predicament")

ask everyone at dinner to share the best
thing that happened to them that day

write three things you like about a
friend on a postcard and send it
anonymously

allow things to unfold in their own good
time

hand down your recipes

reinvent yourself

observe your own observational behavior

make a miniature model

wave out the car's back window

take a poet to lunch

adopt an animal at the zoo

cradle somcone mentally or physically

stake a plant

master painting with acrylics

dye Easter eggs

look before you leap

carefully climb up on a roof

try on all your shoes and donate the uncomfortable ones

glimpse a new horizon

bring food to a needy person

sit quietly and enjoy your own company

call in to a radio talk show

regard another attendee at an event

sketch a tree

do sit-ups

discuss politics, gently

create a pleasing little surprise for your partner

listen to the top 40 songs

scoop up a mass of leaves that have been
floating in a puddle and examine them

cocoon with the family

illustrate every item on a list with
a doodle

scrutinize and manipulate familiar
objects in your immediate
proximity

make art in bed

capture a sentence
uttered by a stranger

curl up, listening to the wind

prove you are right about a word's
meaning or spelling, politely

fuel up for a trip

recount your dreams for someone

make a mini-sculpture out of objects in
the room

watch a painting video with paints and
paper ready 📱

look for the color blue in your surroundings to relax your nervous system

make vegetable juice

start learning a new language with Duolingo

chop your own wood

get rid of something that brings you down or holds you back

rake and replenish the mulch

watch people coming and going, write down three things you notice about each person, then look for patterns

read a print magazine

write a poem as a wedding gift

do a hair mask

pick up the mail

do something that scares you

invent a salad dressing

build a pond in your backyard

eat a meal with mindfulness, making it
   last as long as possible

list the things you wanted to buy but
   didn't

create your own uniform

ask a parent to teach you something

visit a natural wonder

turn your pillow over

talk to the person next to you

call your mother

pretend you are in a zoo

think of something likeable about the
   person you dislike the most

teach a child to read

sit in front of a mirror and draw what
   you see

offer to go out for a coffee run

share a perfect silence

follow a set of footprints

set a physical challenge for yourself

find your sunglasses

make a mini-posy from flowers growing
up out of cracks in the sidewalk

explore a new neighborhood

read the owner's manuals

discover a shortcut on your way home

replace your shopping cart

complete a jigsaw puzzle

plan an atypical Thanksgiving menu

feng shui your home and change your life
by moving 27 objects

perfect your tennis backhand

write the message you want to send in
a bottle

participate in ax throwing

whip up a salad

organize your recipes

watch your handwriting as ink flows out
of the pen

organize a neighborhood get-together

wait for the tide by the shore

name your plants and put their names on their pots

vacuum the inside of the car

make sure the oil tank is full

try something someone else's way

leave a small surprise gift in the refrigerator

train for a hike

create a picture wall

trace a route on a map with a yellow highlighter

hang a suncatcher or prism in a window

thank the trash collector

go out to a marsh with field glasses

test the water with a toe

give yourself permission to leave a retreat, meeting, movie, etc., before it is over

teach yourself to juggle

fill out a survey

teach someone to swim

go to an exercise class

take up yoga

do an ink drawing of your partner or
child

take care of that niggling thing that
surfaced recently

notice the absurdities around you,
especially in a place with a lot of
signs, like an airport

sweep the garage floor

take a plant and move it to the garden

stop and smell the roses

discover the power of stillness

decide to make time for something

spend the first 15 minutes of your day
planning to do something nice for
yourself

dance in the rain

sit on the porch in the evening

compile a list of 50 facts about yourself

share your toys

seek a meaningful and positive mantra or affirmation

begin a new course of learning

bag your groceries

see what you can do blindfolded

become a regular at a coffee shop, food truck, or bookstore and make friends with the staff and other regular customers

imagine the scene of someone finding your message in a bottle

put the cap back on a pen

run in the snow

go on a road trip with friends

replace a missing button with a similar button in a different color

give yourself a gentle pinch to get yourself going

recite your wedding vows

get a little sunburned on your lunch hour

taste test a bottle of possibly expired wine

find the perfect setting on the toaster

reflect on your goals

feel the season bursting around you

redecorate your office door or cubicle wall

bake a giant cookie for someone

rearrange a room for better flow

adopt a shelf at the library and make weekly visits to line up the books

find a place where you can read to the elderly

read your old journals or diaries

put up the storm sashes

make a meal out of whatever you have in your fridge

prep the snowblower

pore over design books

do a rain dance for dry land

drink a glass of water

change the song in your head

pick your own Academy Award winners

paint the insides of closets or cabinets a bright color

open your perception to a bigger worldview

notice the sensation of your pants, socks, or shoes against your skin

nap in the sunshine

focus your attention on remembering someone you have lost

find a religious or spiritual practice that truly works for you

massage your scalp

map the textures in your home

make something you've never tried to make before, like risotto balls listen for the spaces between sounds

let a friend pour their heart out

invent a new pasta sauce

create a picnic using ingredients from a local farmers market

jump rope on one foot

learn how to sew

jump into bed with a good book

watch the sky and wait for a falling star

jot down sentences you like when you read them

try a new fruit or vegetable, such as an ugli fruit

join the volunteer fire department

make a cup using origami and drink water from it

join an outdoor adventure club

make a puppet from a brown paper bag

notice something you always notice, then notice something you never notice invite a loved one to snuggle

make a list with crayons

look at tadpoles in a pond

indulge in some playacting

identify the predicate of a sentence

notice a small gesture

make homemade mustard

identify a common theme in both work
and pleasure that you enjoy

hit the showers

hide a spare key

hang up your coat or jacket

listen to the music of the rain

grow a watermelon

go outside to read your book in the sun

throw your pet a party

join a running club

create an island of being in an island
of doing

put price tags on items for a tag sale

choose a place to live or visit by closing your eyes and pointing to the map

get off the path you have beaten

get in touch with your spiritual side

walk to a bakery and buy yourself a cookie

garden in your backyard

follow the sun

fold a piece of paper in half perfectly

tell yourself a joke

find out the history of a building

explore an unknown street

practice yoga or tai chi outdoors

examine your sewing kit for things you will never use

start tracking your water consumption with a water-tracking app

give the pet a sponge bath

enjoy a relaxed meal

eat the thing you are cooking while
   cooking it

plot your escape route

drop a line to an old friend

drive a post

draw the space surrounding an object,
   not the object itself

make a list of your positive personality
   traits

trim your cat's claws

donate books to those who will benefit
   from and enjoy them

exercise at the office

do something to make yourself smile and
   feel alive and energized

recycle old plastic containers

eat at half speed

discover something you forgot you had

design the purse or wallet of your dreams

delight in the smallest of things

decorate with your favorite things

declare a worry-free day

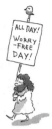

draw something the next time you
    are tempted to photograph
    something

give yourself a new name for the
    next hour

dance the twist

start a mini vegetable garden

dance on the roof, carefully

plan a party for no reason

cut your teeth on a new project

create a personal time capsule to be
    found a century from now

design a retirement community

create art with someone you love

work on your bike

craft a *wabi-sabi* object, which
    is intentionally imperfect,
    impermanent, or incomplete

try to locate an owl in the evening

count your food storage containers and keep only what you need

take your shoes off

cut out paper snowflakes

cook with a new ingredient

make a list of your obsessions

take all the books off the shelves, then put them back in a different order

create the perfect sandwich

finish a knitting project

construct a picture frame

find an object of relaxation that you can carry as a reminder

combine two sauces to make a unique sauce

cleanse your crystals with salt

clear your mind by sitting alone in silence

draw a picture with your eyes closed

decorate a small bushel basket

clear out what isn't useful or beautiful

chronicle your interesting dating escapades

paint a sidewalk mosaic

change what you do in a room to something you don't normally do there

notice the sensation of your body moving through space

change a tire

arrange a tailgate party

read your own tarot cards

draw an optical illusion

celebrate the things you strike off your to-do list

catch up with a friend

check the time and weather in foreign cities ▢

campaign to save the rain forest

call a wise sibling for advice

build an inventory of sounds you detect

write a play for children

brush your teeth with your nondominant
hand

watch a moth fluttering against the
lights

clear the underbrush

browse a secondhand bookstore

do something that improves the world

bring in the mail for elderly neighbors

build a personal altar or shrine

bring a quality of attention and love to
the minute and repetitive aspects of
your commute

perfect a bartending trick

donate a tree to a local park

become an expert thrift store shopper

make a list of your frustrations and how
you might resolve them

be alert to flashes of unexpected beauty
and surprising acts of courage,
compassion, wit, or wisdom

attempt to see something from as many
angles as possible

at the end of the day, note five things you
did for yourself

be an apprentice

ask your partner for a slow dance

do nothing else while drinking hot tea or
coffee

arrange to meet someone at a geographic
halfway point

allow the muscles in your jaw to
relax

allow a yo-yo to unwind itself

admire a straight seam

**celebrate a very tiny occasion,
such as putting on your socks**

act on a generous thought that arises
spontaneously in your heart

tinker with a familiar recipe, like pasta sauce

go to an event with the intent of paying attention to the sounds

make spaghetti sauce without using tomatoes

read a poem by Billy Collins, even if you think you hate poems

learn to restore furniture

dye your hair a crazy color

do a pratfall

read a paper or report aloud before turning it in

reuse packaging

clean out the refrigerator

write down everything you think for the next 20 minutes

come up with a vanity license plate that describes you

volunteer at a local animal rescue center

shred unnecessary, potentially sensitive documents, like receipts with credit card numbers

treat yourself to a romantic dinner for one

clean out a closet

scribble with crayons to music

take an epic bike ride

create a personal recipe book

set up an exercise space in your home

put stuff away

put together a work portfolio

dabble in drawing, watercolor, pastels, oil painting, acrylics, or mixed media

put the patio umbrella away

sneak outside to enjoy some sun

prepare a surprise

make a list of words, then a synonym for each word

improve your relationship with
    your boss

get to know your neighbors

have a playdate

focus on the sensations coming from
    your coffee: the warmth, the steam

find a reliable babysitter

fix a snagged sweater

feel your brain thinking

design your own wallpaper

taste something new

count the shades of a color you see from
    a window

listen to the traffic

do a restorative relaxation yoga pose

use old paper and files as packing
    material

disguise a part of yourself, such as
    your voice, your style, or your
    handwriting, for an hour

explore a college campus

give solace to someone who needs it

practice dribbling a basketball

try on clothes that you think no longer fit
    you, and donate them if they don't

do lanyard lacing

settle a disagreement with a dance-off

offer to braid someone's hair

access a point of stillness at the center of
    your being

introduce yourself to someone you know
    but never speak to

name four things you can hear in
    the room

customize a skateboard

dream up a unique school fundraiser

sit back and enjoy the view

look up how to rig a lean-to in
    the woods

copy a favorite poem

poke around for cat toys under the
    refrigerator

snuggle

move furniture to fully sweep the floor

go bushwalking

prep a big meal

make a list of good hiding places for
    presents

go watch a nearby sporting event

take mail to the mailbox

name the colors in your own box of
    64 crayons

play Simon Says

buy flowers for your kitchen

memorize Hamlet's soliloquy that begins,
    "To be or not to be"

take a lesson in exotic dancing, such as
    belly dancing

put a note in someone's pocket with a list
    of things you like about them

put Velcro strips on something that
     needs it

go on a retreat

memorize a short poem

do the thing you are best qualified to do

put stickers on items to beautify them

open a new jar of peanut butter and draw
     a picture in the smooth top

allow music to transport you

if you're in the passenger
     seat, close your eyes

dispense a single excellent, helpful hint

try one of the specials at a place where
     you always get the same thing

show restraint

open to a blank page and commit to
     writing for 15 minutes

serve at the soup kitchen

build white space into your calendar

watch fish

set the curve on a test

bicycle across town

crack a secret code

sing karaoke

try honey instead of sugar in your coffee

gather your thoughts in peace

create a personal growth journal

roll up the rugs and dance

keep tabs on the neighbors

train your dog to do one trick

double back, walk sideways, or simply
stop altogether and stare at the sky

make a wish with a penny thrown into
a fountain

churn your own butter

make a list of what to take on a trip

watch kids play games

discover the difference between rocks
and minerals

take a slice of pizza to the park

rotate the underwear in the drawer

dance all night

start a bullet/dot journal using special
pens

get physical

count every grain in a pile of rice

get a library card

design an advertising campaign for
a cause you believe in

find the perfect present

feel the rain on your face

put butter on every individual bite of
a muffin or roll

embrace spontaneity

listen to the lulling song of the ocean

service your car

defrost a refrigerator

replace worn shoelaces

flip or turn the mattress

draw a picture of the room you're in

look for something new in a familiar environment, like the walk from your car to your office

invent a themed menu based on your own travels

map out your ideal road trip

dig in the garden until you discover something delightful

find animal tracks

concentrate fully on a food's flavor

risk the possibility of feeling lost and make a journey with no digital guidance

picnic on the fire escape

tighten all the screws in your home

grab a friend and play a game of H-O-R-S-E

alternate bites of different foods

make a list of your driver's license and credit card numbers in case you lose your wallet

retract a lie

make a list of what to do when the power goes out

skip stones across a lake

take a natural history tour of your area

finish off the leftovers

deejay with a turntable

study facial expressions

do headstone rubbings of graves

beautify the basement

refinish your floors

collect 100 affirmations

eat out on the porch

reenact a scene from your favorite movie

answer your cat's questions

consider what you would like to be
reincarnated as

smell the spices in the spice cabinet and
toss ones with no scent

marinate the grill food

practice ear wiggling

learn orienteering

find old love letters

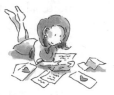

switch seasonal coats in the closet

stain a piece of furniture

banter with a cashier

scrutinize whatever written information
is available

play ping-pong with a friend or against
a wall

look back on your life's passions and
find connections

determine a purpose for something you
want to undertake as well as what the
outcome may be

invite your grandmother on an outing

sow seeds

learn to purl

teach an interested senior citizen
   something on the computer

do a painting on butcher paper

knead bread dough by hand

think of a way to make some extra
   cash

change the quality of your thoughts to be
   more positive, loving, and happy

assist someone who's struggling

make a list of volunteer activities that
   you would enjoy and to which you
   would bring a special skill

involve one or more of your senses in
   a novel context (e.g., eat with
   earplugs in)

pick a single sound and listen for it

reunite sock pairs

make an I Wish list, then take action

break into song and dance

ask a Ouija board some questions

convert a room or garage into a private study

write a letter to your third-grade teacher, positive or negative

strike up a conversation with a stranger

put on noise-canceling headphones and sit in silence for 30 minutes

do yard work

learn a few words in the language(s) of your ancestors

discover where your mind wanders

help a friend

write a message or design in the condensation on car windows

explore the things that you accidentally missed

play crazy eights

catch a fish with your bare hands

stack a woodpile

use a tongue scraper

get better and better at things you
    do well

stake and train a fruit tree

brush up on grammar rules

throw away old or unmeaningful
    Christmas ornaments

get kids to do the activity for which they
    have the longest attention span

tell someone the single most valuable
    thing you have learned

fold socks and stockings into thirds or
    halves, then halve again and stand on
    end in a drawer

go to an event where you won't know
    anyone and see how it feels

have a conversation with Siri

learn tae kwon do

find a place for that thing that's always in
    the way

see your morning routine as
    performance art

find a quiet spot to observe

list ideas for future projects

take something that you see every day
    and try to see it in a different light

look around a pet store

make a list of things to try in your life

get old ideas out of your mind by
    reframing them

study the teachings of a sage or holy
    person

come up with funny messages for
    valentine heart candies

plan a class or office prank

knead thoughts

write a play

spin a top

watch the cat bathe itself

do something superfast or super slow

take the focus off yourself and feel love and compassion for someone else

build a nest and see if a bird comes

focus on one thing and look for the sacred in it, Shinto-style

travel across the room taking two steps forward and one step back

play in the dirt

separate the recycling for the garbage pickup

relax your neck, jaw, and tongue

plan a new adventure for Sunday

impart knowledge to a silent audience, like a tree or a snail

bullet-point your life history

call to a bird or owl

design a public space

triple-tie your shoelaces

pay attention to the room tone or the barely audible noises that make up a background sense of quiet improvise an air freshener using natural ingredients from outdoors

pack a picnic for the beach

remove one piece of furniture from a room

observe a spider spinning its web

explore with friends

create a sniglet, an invented word for a concept that does not have a name

mix Valentine's Day and Easter candy

create a painting with stippling (small dots)

floss your teeth while doing the floss dance

make a list of things to sell at a garage sale

loosen too-tight lids in the cabinet and fridge

take a nap in tall grass

learn how to pack a suitcase efficiently

harvest what you have planted

watch the sand in an hourglass

unkink muscles with a foam roller

try a new food or ingredient found at a
farmers market

thank items you're donating or disposing
of for all they have given you

make your own cheese

shorten your to-do list

figure out the telescope

contemplate your place in the universe

hunt for interesting rocks

identify all the state capitals

play a game of four square

practice your free throws

have your palm read

schedule that appointment you've been
putting off

give a gift anonymously

patch the driveway

get someone to play chess with you

learn braille

focus the next hour on taste

donate canned goods; toss the expired ones

read a novel aloud with a friend

descale the kettle

do nine-part breathing—inhale three short breaths, exhale three, pause for three

pick up the dry cleaning

create tessellations

invent a personal prayer of thanks

learn correct pronunciations

make a list of things to do once the snow melts

eat food blindfolded

picture a scene in your mind's eye and feel it in your body

do a shoutout for a friend

string popcorn

fill the saltshaker

bathe in the sounds around you and
find a point of silence within

fill a jug or pitcher with a colorful
bouquet of flowers

write letters to people in places you've
moved from and send them, or not

look at something stationary for two
solid minutes, then look away and
jot down what you remember

plan your Halloween costume

cast a horoscope

draw on paper place mats

putter about the house

donate a working computer to a school
or senior center

rock out in the car

do your own basic car maintenance

espouse a theory

notice the rhythms of the gym

tweeze your eyebrows

go for a Sunday drive

devise a vocabulary quiz

beg someone for details,
an answer, or a look at
something

clean up the garden

create and name a new color

clean a favorite piece of jewelry

recycle jewelry

look for shadows

learn needlepoint

put a new picture on your desk at work

spoil someone rotten

make a list of things to do in wintertime

run with your dog or child

invent a word game

go fishing

find a nice rock and paint it to look like
a pet

learn to pot plants

do the thing you think you cannot do

do an impression of a friend or frenemy

buy a specialized dictionary and learn
the terms in it

have an eating contest

build something out of wood

fillet a fish

ask questions that others will enjoy
answering

dawdle in the present tense

ask for recommendations of things to do
wherever you are

act with a local repertory theater

arrange a platter of fruit

draw little pictures for someone's
amusement

find a book set in a place you'd like to
travel to

learn one good card trick

feel yourself becoming drowsy

admire someone's originality

stick googly eyes on everything

listen to the lowing of cattle in a nearby field

stop to take three deep breaths rather than rushing on to the next thing

add a touch of charades to your conversation

draw, which is all about slowing down and deep looking

sip some hot water with lemon

join a pickleball league

go barefoot

create a lost pet poster featuring a unicorn and post it in your neighborhood

volunteer at a zoo

choose a person to secretly follow until they enter a space you cannot enter

take the road less traveled

make a list of things to do in the fall

create a rebus

take a moment to notice some basic
     sensations, like the ebb and flow of
     your breath

pretend to be an actor

hide pet toys and check later to see if
     they've been found

discover really interesting things about
     words that you never knew before

plant a metaphorical seed for something
     you want to grow

listen to some new music

imagine that you believe six impossible
     things are possible

look through schoolwork from when you
     were young

list all the restaurants you go to most
     often and add a brand-new one to the
     list for next time

deconstruct an artist's style

learn a new word and use it

put pretty shells in a jar

get your family out the door to work and school on time

take a selfie with your pet

drive to the mountains

analyze what kind of thoughts your mind produces

decide what you wish someone would ask you about

have a pillow fight

make a flavored lemonade with thyme or rosemary

make or visit a butterfly house

plant daffodils and tulips

clean the golf clubs

toss out junk food

pay close attention to the bark on trees

make an ankle bracelet

attend a community event

get a hot stone massage

dig into the source of a word's meaning

find the perfect patch of grass to sit on at the park

prune a bush

imagine going to space with the people in your immediate vicinity

feel the power of lifting a weight

learn to use a loom

make a list of things to do in the area for your guests

trace the shape of an intricate object

create a nom de plume

carry someone over a puddle

run the vacuum attachment over the dog

play pin the tail on the donkey

count smiles in the room

make flavored ice cubes using mint and lemon or lime

go to a yoga class

delight someone

play I Spy in alphabetical order

pause as you eat by putting down your
utensils between bites

discover inner wealth

come up with a gratitude prayer to say
before a meal

make vanilla pudding and put it in an
empty mayonnaise jar

come up with a title for a new book

swing on a swing set

complete all the tasks on your day's to-do
list

adventure around town, exploring places
you've never been

color outside the lines

collect rocks of all one shape

pass along a good book to someone

color walls with crayons before
   wallpapering

invent five friendly nicknames

perfume dresser drawers with hotel
   soaps

stage an unexpected performance in
   a public place

paint one fingernail a wild color

blanch crudités

instigate a fun plan

jog along a waterfront

feed pigeons at a park

eat snow ice cream

video chat with faraway family or friends 📱

make a snow globe

tie back your hair

draw with children

make a list of fun but unlikely things to
   do after work, then do one

skateboard

find what that smell is

learn to properly remove a mango from its skin

go into the countryside after a rain

make amends for that thing you did—you know the one

call a gym and ask for a free day pass

fill every notebook you own with new ideas

sing at the top of your lungs with the windows open

fluff up the pillows

play basketball

neaten and clean up paint boxes and paintbrushes

test a proverb, such as "a bird in the hand is worth two in the bush"

jump up and click your heels together

leave the office for lunch

play a Tibetan singing bowl to relax

unscrew a jar on the first try

your responses

sprinkle lavender essential oil in your
sleeping area

buy environmentally friendly light bulbs

sort laundry and put it away

help your favorite teacher after school

blend into your surroundings

derive pleasure from knowing something

write a message in code

treat yo'self

watch a leaf descend

research how to force spring bulbs to
blossom

listen to a recording of dolphins or
whales singing

go jogging at sunset

build a model with a child

eat on the floor Japanese-style

visit a museum about a topic you have no
   interest in and see what happens

carol with candles

talk to the locals

request the pleasure of a dance

make a list of things that money can't buy

patchwork a quilt

get down on the ground for a different
   view

play beanbag toss

create a nice picture

listen to a guru speak on YouTube

pretend you are in a movie

lighten another's burden

start a game of 20 Questions

invent something

organize the junk drawer

store bags inside one large bag

take a hot/cold contrast shower,
    quickly changing the temperature
    from hot to cold and back again

dangle a fishing line into water

follow a river path

**find someone who wants
    their hair brushed**

imagine your road less traveled

fast for a day

learn to play the guitar

climb rock piles

do a needlework project

compose magnetic poetry on the
    refrigerator

change the pictures in your wallet

go stargazing

play rock paper scissors

discover a secret of nature

ask yourself trivia questions from
    a board game

draw a picture of the building across the street

wake up a half hour earlier and take a walk

change your jogging or walking route

dance alone for relaxation

correct all the spelling and grammatical errors on everything you see

drive up and down the main street of town looking for a lost pet

find a cool place to stay overnight, like a submarine or lighthouse

visit a sculpture park

volunteer for parks and recreation programs

make a list of things that have been bugging you

tap trees for sap

study servicepeople—look at what they are wearing, their expressions, and what they are looking at

make corner bookmarks

smile at people in other cars

sand wood

have lunch with a friend
(but not your phone)

twitch your nose like a bunny

make a list of funny Truth or Dare
questions

visit an escape room

hatch a plan

equip a guest room with toiletries and
a robe

pick a single perfect wildflower from
a field of many

smell old books

make fondue

make a new kind of ice cream float

cure or honey-bake a ham

keep a list of words to look
up in dictionaries

design a miracle

know that resting is also restorative if
you cannot sleep

think of how you can be lovable to
someone in particular

include a surprise in a kid's lunch or
snack: a picture, cartoon, or note

take your pulse

change your voice mail message 📱

make and color a map

begin a 1,000-piece puzzle

finish a home improvement project

orient your movements to a distant
object on the horizon

watch bunnies play

enjoy the silence

go sledding on the lawn with a plastic sled

make your own jigsaw puzzle

museum-hop

read a mystery book from your childhood

skid across a wood floor in socks

clean out the freezer

breathe out the negative, breathe in
the positive

create a new neural pathway by walking
backward up the stairs

chart a soundwalk, a walk that has points
of interest based on sounds

go for a five-mile run

plan Halloween costumes that use only
one color

squeeze stress balls with both hands and
both feet

beg someone's pardon

find a pure white rock

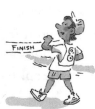

walk for a cure

knit an outfit for your dog
or cat

decorate a room to make it look bigger

put worn or single socks in the rag bin

play a game of paintball

arrive early for a dinner out or a meeting and observe your surroundings

divide perennials

find exactly the right words

dawdle over coffee

retreat to a spa

watch people interact

try someone else's meal, with their permission

put a message in a bottle and float it out on a body of water

think less, do more

save your fruit seeds and plant them in public spaces

do the splits—or a split, depending on where you grew up

pause at a window

open a drawer and sort the contents

secure the lid of a container

buy a doughnut

close your eyes and think about all the good things that happened today

transform a routine into a Zen moment with mindfulness

make the bed

smoke a turkey

extract blackheads

name as many uses as you can think of for a toothpick

imagine buying all the things you desire and figure out where you would put them

roll around in your office chair

swim laps

build cat walkways in your house

sort through makeup and throw out old products

play Mother, may I?

seize the day

monitor the involuntary and intentional
    sounds you emit

help at a nursing home or senior center

become part of the silence

recycle greeting cards as bookmarks

go behind the scenes

explore back roads

pick a route that takes twice the time

display a favorite book

make an I Spy jar for a child

catch someone smiling to themselves

ask a new friend if they have a favorite
    color

decipher new words from their roots

brighten the view of something you look
    at every day

go to a town meeting and speak your
    mind

shoot pool

eat cookies and milk in the car

convene a power breakfast at a local
   diner

bark at passing dogs

download a meditation app
   and use it

improvise a dinner

**point north from where
   you are**

create a story using shadow puppets

look at your phone usage monitor, and
   vow to reduce that time

put money into an adventure fund

play hot potato

make a list of the successes in your life

raid the refrigerator

decoupage

assemble materials to do a new kind
   of art

sharpen a pencil

invent and celebrate your own holiday

lean against a corner of the wall to massage your back

create a new dish

disconnect from all the chatter

consider five ways to make small talk with strangers

picture what it would be like to live in a clutter-free space

watch an ASMR video 📱

try a new exercise program

enter a poetry slam

make your own candy

hit golf balls

figure out the suitcase lock combination

search your soul

practice lucid dreaming

cook double portions of your favorite recipe and freeze half

start over

break trail in the snow

rock in a chair

go train-spotting

turn regular sentences into poetry

paint a portrait

emancipate a trapped bug

notice the quality of the light

remove winter clothes from storage

learn to play the harmonica

make some firewood into feather sticks
with a pocketknife

do a logroll down a hill

browse through an antique store

go for a short hike at a wilderness park

make a list of the places you've traveled

watch the river flow while standing on
a bridge

connect disparate ideas

count how many people in your vicinity
are on phones

draw up a will

chew on life's big questions

pierce your ears

meet an old friend for coffee

take bets on when your food is going to arrive at a restaurant or deli

piece a quilt

learn dictionary lookup skills

memorize two good jokes

wear two different earrings

distract your partner

accept this minute as an unrepeatable miracle

find the perfect pastime

create sandcastle ruins for a prehistoric civilization

declare peace

fix bent glasses

collect kindling

refill the bird feeder

I DECLARE!!

pretend you're vacationing on
    a tropical island

sing "The Star-Spangled Banner"

flip the sofa and chair cushions

color inside the lines

dangle participles

meditate while polishing silver

philosophize

take notes for your autobiography

create a new compost pile in your
    backyard

smudge your home with sage, juniper,
    or cedar

blow up balloons

show initiative

make a list of the languages you are
    aware of

install a Medical ID app on your phone in
    case of emergency

create your own weight lifting workout

lie down on the floor and do a progressive
muscle relaxation

plan new outfits or ways to wear old
clothes

climb into a hammock

write a manifesto

form hypotheses

watch a happy animal

make a piecrust from scratch

talk to your kids about what they're
looking at on their phones

create a new dip

do an ab exercise

hobnob with the cool crowd

concentrate with all your being on
whatever attracts your attention

absorb an impression

volunteer at the school cafeteria

look for reflections

put your clothes away

keep everyone up-to-date on the weather forecast

install carbon monoxide and smoke detectors

fix a snafu

use a magnifying glass to look at something from nature

designate a place for each category of object in your home, like seasonal clothing

sharpen an ax

choose how to live the next year of your life

stand for 20 minutes for every sitting hour

lubricate door hinges

create best-of lists

deliver hope

let off steam

design lingerie

toss bread to the ducks on a pond

shadowbox your opponent

recycle the junk mail

play hangman

watch an inchworm through a
    magnifying glass

make a list of the different kinds of tools
    you know how to use

eat honey straight from the jar

shower and shave

find a pond or stream and lose
    yourself watching dragonflies,
    fish, and frogs

plant herbs in window boxes

donate some new books to
    a nursing home

stretch

scribble ideas on scraps of paper

go for a 20-minute walk, no matter
    the weather

return that thing you borrowed

rehash the day

buy a Powerball ticket

wiggle your ears

figure out how to ask a question on
WolframAlpha

redesign a workspace

visualize your goals and success

turn your own name into a chant

collect seashells

ask people about what they are reading

list names and page numbers of favorite
recipes inside cookbook covers

intervene in an unnecessary argument

**crouch in a garden and watch
the wildlife**

notice an animal, flower, or tree

read in bed before sleep

saw wood

synchronize the clocks

meditate before bedtime on what you'd like to dream about

tutor a child

register new voters

read visual dictionaries to learn the parts of things

bicycle to and from errands

remove dead leaves from the houseplants

do pull-ups

draw graffiti with a pencil

create a dream catcher with found objects

make a list of smoothies you want to make

ventilate the house

come up with nail polish color names

walk very, very slowly across a room

expand the world of what you eat

catch somebody singing in their car and share a laugh with them experience the place you are in

get started making soup

lift a fingerprint easily with baby powder
    and tape

memorize some Dr. Seuss

ponder a distant horizon and imagine
    what's going on there

proofread what you have written

create a new college major

prepare mashed potatoes without
    a single lump

sketch food

climb stairs until your heart pounds

run errands on foot

practice Ujjayi breath, breathing with
    your lips closed and making sounds
    like Darth Vader

send a homemade postcard

conduct a self-interview

start a gratitude list

refuel a chain saw, a lawn mower, or the car

refill the toilet paper

burn a yellow candle to promote calmness

wait outside a church when there's a wedding

do only what a child wants to do

index a book

play catnip games with your cat

dine outdoors

scratch an itch

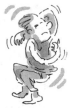

hand-deliver a message

shred an old textbook into confetti

do five-second breathing meditations at the end of each paragraph you read

take the first step in just one of your "million-dollar" ideas

mist indoor plants

freeze colored sugar water or juice in ice cube trays

make a list of new TV shows to try out

frost a perfectly smooth cake

try a new kind of plant milk

sand and oil garden and toolbox tools

fix an item you love instead of
    replacing it

listen to the crash of waves on the
    rocks

go clamming

learn to paint with oils

offer to babysit

do a little work on Sunday so you can
    sit outside for a couple of hours on
    beautiful Monday

join a health club

read a kid's comic book collection

learn how to make a sun compass or
    improvise a magnetic compass

put a master plan into action

create an inner sieve, with happiest thoughts at the surface and heaviest thoughts dropping away

go on a news fast

choose a papier-mâché project

do the robot dance

remember to look up

clean out the fireplace

put on funny socks

learn a specific self-defense move

learn the hula or the mambo

plan a large project with tasks and milestones

help a disabled person

keep a list of things that are subtly changing around you

hold a BOGO sale

design a memorable day

catch a fish and throw it back in

make your own seasoned salt

wash the potholders

come up with a solution to a
   work problem

hunt for dropped pennies

throw a paper airplane out a high window

record your wildlife sightings with
   a nature app

invent a new sport

teach a child the alphabet, numbers,
   shapes, or colors

eat a healthy meal

sit in deep shade

create your own pizza

share a passage from a book

write down every new idea you have

set a mousetrap

discover where you are on the letter
   carrier's route

read the notes in the back of the book
that match up with the pages
you read

order or buy some new stationery

put your lawn mower back in its place

create a new breakfast cereal

burn a brown candle to protect pets and
solve home problems

take an elevator friend to lunch

perfect your golf swing

set up an art stash with markers, paper,
crayons, scissors, tape, etc.

participate in an open-mic night

put together a traveling art kit

prepare a salad using 20 different
ingredients

name your home

improve your posture

make sure the gas tank is full

get to know the night sky and watch it
change with the seasons

leave a romantic message

focus on the happy encounters
around you

hang a spoon on your nose

shape up your abdominals

do an arm workout using a heavy
household object, like a cast
iron pan

put the ice/snow scraper in the car or
take it out

design your own tattoo

give yourself an egg white facial

make a list of everything you want to do
before your next birthday

fill out an organ donor card and a
living will

do an eye-palming exercise for relaxation
and clearer vision

after a flash of lightning, count the
      seconds until you hear thunder;
      divide the total by five to know how
      many miles away the storm is

write your own epitaph

consider the power of prayer

volunteer as a scorekeeper

decide to let it go

use your gift cards and gift certificates

dance in the moonlight

throw out pencils with worn-out erasers

compile a list of botanical specimens

tell a kid you like what they are wearing

climb a stone wall

study a pair of hands

begin a new breakfast ritual

spend time in an ashram

become a bird-watcher

sneak a late-night snack

bake a dessert

inhale the scent of the grass

adopt a rescue animal

sharpen the scissors

write to an enemy you are ready to stop
fighting with

send a letter to the artist you most
admire

interview a person you admire

winterize the garden

find a place of your own to master the art
of doing nothing

whittle a walking stick

ask for help

try looking at something familiar as
if you'd never seen it before while
waiting in a long line

learn the art of digital drawing

seek out free wildlife viewing spots
near you

weave a lattice-top pie

seek awe in the sea—birds diving, fish leaping

wave to the neighbors

make a list of everything you own that you want to get rid of

wave at kids on school buses

take a meandering walk with no destination

water the plants

search for the end of a rainbow

watch rain slide off the roof

rig a pulley system

look at snowflakes close up

wash all the windows

reorganize the linen closet

wash a head of lettuce leaf by leaf

remember the name of somebody or something after it's been on the tip of your tongue for days

warm your pajamas before you get
   in them

read an entire book in a cozy corner
   of a bookstore

take a forest walk with a person versed
   in flora or fauna

create a new board game

put things on high shelves when there
   is no use for them

walk to work

put something together

walk through an orchard

write a love story

watch a fly

walk at half speed

do something selfless

visit the lesser known, off-the-beaten-
   path art museums

build a miniature golf course

visit an art gallery

practice pulling a tablecloth off a table
without breaking anything

prepare for takeoff

watch an earth-moving truck at work

create a six-word memoir about yourself

practice for the SAT

turn the lights down low

turn over to even out your tan

get a good explanation

turn down the covers

find or create the perfect card for
someone

turn a source of irritation into an
opportunity to be mindful

feel the peace of old trees

try an herbal remedy

walk on stilts

play the sport of the season

transform your daily life into drawings

perform a spiritual inventory of your life

touch your tongue to your nose

create a "blackout poem" from a
newspaper article

get rid of products from health crazes
you no longer pursue

offer a cup of coffee at an unexpected
time

time a Walk/Don't Walk light

mend a hole in your pocket

tie a slipknot

watch seals being fed at a zoo via
live cam 📱

create a replica of a Minecraft sword
using materials you have on hand

master a new gadget

take a pair of jeans you never wear and
recycle them into something new

look up something you have never quite
understood or have always wanted to
know more about

do a little extra work each day so you can take Friday off

light a dark corner

imitate a funny person

teach your hobby

remember something you abandoned over the past year—a project or an idea—and think about restarting the venture

invite a new kid to join you for lunch

talk yourself out of that thing you don't have to do

have an elegant tea party

take yourself to lunch

take out the trash, metaphorically

paint a piece of pottery

practice burping

play music loud enough to make someone say, "Turn it down!"

take a selfie with a squirrel 📱

make a list of everything you keep
"just in case" and save it to review in
six months

take note of the words around you

notice where the pressure points are
from the seat you are sitting on

take in your physical environment
carefully, then go to a different room
and sketch or write about it

go for a run on city streets at night,
when they are empty of traffic

take down the holiday decorations

go back to the drawing board

survey the scene

give away something you never liked

**surround yourself with
things you love**

get up and walk around

surprise someone with their
favorite sandwich

file your nails

submit a suggestion that saves money for your company

get out of the doghouse

stroll through a state park

stretch your toes as far apart as you can

create a mural

stop thinking about how you wish it could be and realize how good you've got it

learn how to make a great cup of coffee

go to a spinning class

stop at a turnout to appreciate the view

watch the pet watch something

steam your outfit for tonight or tomorrow

try a new coffee shop

stay up all night talking

make your kitchen the most comfortable room in the house

start keeping chickens

figure out the meaning of life for yourself

stare into the eyes of someone you love for exactly four minutes

finish the Sunday crossword puzzle

stand on your head

do an unpleasant task right now rather than worry about it

find new ways to charm your mate

sponsor a child in need

make a list of five things you're grateful for

split the housework

take a large magnet to the beach to search for coins

split a quarter cord of wood

pick a room to retreat to for listening to music, puttering, or looking through books

start a bucket list

make an exploration list for your life

perform a random act of kindness

ask a museum guard to tell you the funniest thing he or she's seen happen

sort through old printed photographs

feed a squirrel

learn a new cure to stop the hiccups

sort the sock drawer by color

listen to the clock tick

sit down with your partner, make a list of a few things you have been meaning to do, and set a date for the first one

examine the living things under a rock

request a song to sing

empty the toaster tray

shop in a brick-and-mortar store for something you normally buy online

dust the tops of all the light bulbs in the lamps

shave a peach

drive around the neighborhoods to see
the Christmas lights

share an umbrella

dig out an old yearbook

sew a handmade doll

develop your signature dish

set the timer on the coffee maker

study with your phone in another room
and note how you feel

set off on a ramble

develop a self-improvement program

set aside some books you want to read

compose a mash-up of your favorite
movie plots

set an old chair out in the garden

commit to improving something
that you do

send the laundry out

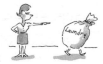

carry a notebook or
sketchbook to an art gallery

send flowers to your best friend for no
particular reason

make a list of everything in your handbag
and/or wallet

send an RSVP

camp out on a beach

select a tiny plant or flower for your desk

put a maraschino cherry on someone's
dessert

see the good in a situation

go on a neighborhood adventure

try to write a dictionary definition and
see how it compares to the real
definition

do the right thing

open a door for others

sculpt a figure out of clay, wood, or stone

close your eyes and say goodbye to each
issue that's on your mind

savor a view

check out the haircuts on the train

run your first mile

create a pantomime dance to a favorite song

run through the sprinkler at night

find a patch of shade

run outside to see the birds or the moon

create a mosaic

read a guilty pleasure novel

restore an old house

clean out the detritus in your backpack or purse

reorganize your work area

be a stabilizing force for someone else

rent a bicycle built for two

balance a spinning Frisbee

remember where you put the gifts you bought early

assemble a portfolio of your art

remember and plan for an anniversary

try talking as fast as an auctioneer

appreciate the reflection, creativity, and renewal that solitude can offer

refashion a vintage necklace

rediscover a simple pleasure

recall a past life

make a list of emergency numbers

rearrange the rearrangement

look for old words and phrases in a 100-year-old dictionary

declare the intention to speak only what is truthful, helpful, and kind

practice hypnosis

read something spiritual

go on a photo safari

run a mile, singing to yourself the whole time

reach out to others

rake the yard

start a garden from scratch

raise your ecological consciousness

plan a hypothetical wedding

put one noodle on each tine of the fork

keep a list of nice things people have said
to you or about you

put an offering in the collection plate

design a line of toys

put all your books on the floor and ask of
each, "Does it spark joy?"

work on a political campaign

pursue your passion

try to identify sounds with your eyes
closed

pull out the kiddie pool and use it

let down your ponytail

provide a hot breakfast on a chilly
morning

finish a drawing

propose a special project

find an object from your childhood and
   turn it into a piece of artwork

preserve a leaf

enjoy the scenery

look at light and shadow in different
   works of art

draw a perfectly straight line without
   a ruler

practice Christmas cookie recipes

learn to make sushi

pore over your favorite art books

make a list of all your important
   documents and where they are

ponder the universe

take a lunch order

polish the silver

do a laundry load of whites

play What if I had a million dollars?

change the order in which you do things

plan your exercise for the next day

decorate a room for the upcoming holiday

place your order at the butcher

stare into the dog's eyes for a full minute

pick the restaurant

people-watch at the mall

peer into shop windows

pause for tea and sweets

read books written by authors from your hometown

part your hair on the opposite side

stare into your own eyes for a full minute

pare down the stuff in your wallet

paint in the middle of the night

create a menu for a restaurant

leave flowers on a neighbor's doorstep

pack for an adventure

observe what other people photograph

notice when you feel most awake

negotiate a great price

name three things you can touch or feel
  in the room

memorize your solo

pause and savor any insights, ideas,
  pictures, or sensations you gain while
  reading

memorize a poem that relaxes you

play a complete game of Monopoly

look up "walking meditation"
  and try it out 📱

measure your body fat

**make a list of all your
  favorite things about someone**

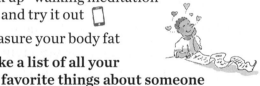

master the art of ventriloquism

read every word on the menu

make two small changes

write a love poem

make someone you care about happy

watch a field being plowed

make real peanut butter

do something outrageous or out of
    character for you

make Christmas cookies

build a house of cards

make as much sound as possible

look out into the far horizon and follow
    a cloud

talk to the driver

paint with watercolors

locate a wall stud

pretend you are an explorer from
    another hemisphere

list the things your parents said they
    would tell you when you're older

play a practical joke

paint an art car

observe how many people in one room
    are staring at a phone

list 100 priceless moments in your life

notice things that may come in handy later

line up beautiful books on a mantelpiece

make the garden plan

lie in the sun and watch autumn leaves fall

learn how to load a backpack efficiently

lick the filling out of a Twinkie

follow a map to its edges

let the rhythm of waves or the wind rock you into calmness

find your reading glasses

leap off a swing onto grass or sand

explore a junkyard

leave funny notes in library books

discover a secret country lane or a peaceful bend in a river

pack your rucksack with a day's supplies

complete a fitness goal

learn what is in the attic

change your handwriting

make a list of all the things you would like to know about someone

build a LEGO city

go to a spa for a treatment

work some Latin into your conversation, such as *tempus fugit*

learn a language in your sleep by playing a recording

leaf through a thesaurus

lie on the grass and look up at the sky

come up with a project for a Kickstarter campaign

begin a new journal of things that make you happy

jump as many stairs as possible

seek out silver linings

invite friends to high tea

introduce a new houseplant

install a dog or cat door

walk behind someone in a crowded place
to see how they cut through the crowd

imagine your mental garbage being
carted away

illustrate your wall calendar

get a goldfish and a goldfish bowl

identify your own biases

find the misplaced keys

create a mental oasis

feel the heat of the sun while sitting
in a car

hug a tree

hop over a log on a bike

hold the elevator for someone

host an international-themed potluck

lie under a ceiling fan and watch the
blades turn

hire someone to wash all the windows

hike a great park

help the helpless

have dinner delivered

illustrate a memory

have breakfast three times in a day

greet the sunrise

imagine you are completely free from the demands and limitations imposed by work, family, and the outside world

make a list of all the things you want to do this spring

go swimming at night

take a Jazzercise class

go someplace warm

go see the oldest person you know

add an unusual item to the shopping list

plan a flash mob event

go off the grid for a day

write the beginning or ending to a play

go downtown with friends

give someone a second chance

write an op-ed

get really into exercise and yoga

gaze at the heavens

gather the neighbors and plant
a community garden

practice that skill that has always
eluded you

frolic in the snow

listen to the cat drink

frame a picture

follow your childhood dream

hang stuff up if your drawers are
overflowing

get rid of or hide things that distract
your attention

fly a kite

flip through magazines at a newsstand

fix up furniture scratches

join a group tour

fix something

eat only with your hands

create an indestructible pet toy

finish an entire word search book

choose a new creative project to work on

look for bookmarks in old books

go home for lunch

volunteer at a school

find inspiration in a work of art

make a list of all the things you know
    how to do

file your taxes early

take the price tag off

establish an exercise routine

film the dog drinking in slo-mo

establish a writing habit

pretend to be a travel writer

engage in small talk

make some homemade play dough

embroider a tablecloth

look for mistakes in a print
    newspaper

learn to make stained glass

plant a rose garden

do a laughing meditation

look through old photo albums

embark on a road trip

list all the silly things you've done for
    money

eavesdrop on public transportation

learn a new language 10 minutes at
    a time

use chopsticks to eat your lunch

get your eyeglasses adjusted

eat under the stars at dusk

go camping by yourself

drive to the fanciest neighborhood in town and go for a walk among the mansions

decide what you want to write about

eat in the living room by the fire

create a memorable ritual

eat an exotic fruit or untried vegetable

cook a vegan meal

put a log on the fire

dwell in the feeling of a nice cool breeze

go on a nature hunt

dust off the fine china

do the one thing you really want to do

drop your tongue to the bottom of your mouth, relaxing your face

make a list of all the symbols you see

attend a city or town council meeting

clean your jewelry

drink tea slowly

clean one dirty window

paint a picture good enough to hang on the wall

check the faces of departing moviegoers in an attempt to determine the quality of the film

notice the play of the shadows

watch a video on how to do The Hustle 📱

eat all your spinach

drink coffee from a delicate porcelain cup

dream up a new prank

draw your vacation pictures instead of taking photos

doze in the sun

donate toys to an organization at Christmas

look at license plates, bumper stickers, and scenery

research how to build a house with Habitat for Humanity

document a view as it changes through the seasons

suggest an activity you want to do and give your partner the option of joining you or not

donate the china if you don't use it

do something you will want to brag about

draw in your head

do a somersault underwater

do Pilates roll ups

put ink on your index finger and draw fingerprint creatures

go grocery shopping for someone

do everything for the next hour with your less dominant hand

divide up the errands

dissect a raspberry

dance with your pet

discover what you want from your
   solitary moments

read a guide on money management

discover new meaning through reflection

clean out the car trunk

dine by moonlight

make a list of all the places you want
   to visit

diagram a task you do every day,
   step-by-step

take a hot bath, followed by a really cold
   shower

have a day of detox

pick up litter and put it where it belongs

determine the one thing in life you want
   most

invent a new food combination

drink a tall glass of milk

deepen your observational powers

eat a food associated with the comforts of childhood

decorate your backpack

create your own maze on paper or in a yard

decorate paper plates

iron the cloth napkins

draw inspiration from your surroundings

cut a labyrinth

cultivate your sense of wonder

create something new out of something old

crash a wedding

crack open a window for ventilation

cozy up with a book

count how many yellow things you see

cook something only you would appreciate

consult a psychic

dance to zydeco

create a mandala drawing

learn to match beats

pierce your own ears with self-piercing
    earrings

learn how to lasso

confide in your best friend

watch the moonrise

concoct a secret formula for a line of
    cosmetics

try a new cereal

concentrate on the sounds of the
    backyard

make a list of all the jobs you have had
    and write a short paragraph on what
    you remember about them

compliment a stranger

make your home secure

communicate with your pet

figure out the centigrade equivalent of
    the temperature

tidy up a room in one fell swoop

combine different mustards on a hotdog

collect your family's recipes

collapse in giggles

start a fad

collaborate on a snowman

plan a graduation party

coin a name for a new generation

keep a list of each day's highs

clip your toenails

go to a playground and play on all
the equipment

clean off your desk

design a greeting card

collect and turn in cans and bottles for
the deposit money

dance a waltz

clean and prep the grill

devise your own trail name

cut up your credit cards

clean all the windows

watch a downpour

choreograph a modern dance

do something nice without being asked

choose to notice things that others
    do not

build a gym for your cat

choose the slowest route, not the fastest

cheer up a lonely person

check your reflection in a mirror

have a nosh

draw a tattoo on your arm with a pen

find a new use for an old bridesmaid
    dress

chat up the receptionist

make a list of all the fun things you have
    done on vacation

chase the shadow of a high-flying bird

try a new genre of book

celebrate an arcane holiday

catch the last rays of sun

put a childhood talent to use in solving an adult challenge

schedule nap time if you lost sleep last night

carve a soap

capture the oddities of your mind on paper

bury your nose in the cat's fur

bundle up to gaze at the stars

brush the dog

learn flag signals

bring your mind back to real time

check for split ends

bring someone soup when they are sick

bring home a surprise from a bakeshop

break out the tennis racket

bow to the sunset

bounce a ripe cranberry

check to see if the fruit is ripe and ready
   to pick

blow the wrapper off a paper straw

bike to work

keep a bedside journal and write as soon
   as you wake up

befriend a squirrel in the yard or park

learn to make rope

become one with your work

do a kindness for a stranger

pick a painting and turn it into a story

change the oil in a car

make an envelope

create a little signal that only your
   partner knows

ask a Magic 8-Ball some questions

lock the door

use a creative metaphor

put on clothes straight from the dryer

train a dog in obedience

catch an ocean breeze

note the empty shelf spots in your grocery store and see what's in demand

take a hot bath by candlelight

tell someone that you love them

learn the difference between stalagmites and stalactites

take something you love to work for show-and-tell

help a community rebuild after a disaster

study the Tao and Confucius

explore the paint swatches at a hardware store

light a green candle to heal energies and bring luck and prosperity

catch a few fireflies in a jar and use it for table lighting

practice a firm handshake

become aware of the pavement in front of you

spin a plate on a stick

beautify your town

spend an hour in silence

beat a personal record

spend a day in the countryside with a sketchbook

bask in the sunshine

join #The100DayProject 📱

look for evidence of ghosts

play in autumn leaves

balance on tiptoe

pay attention to the gaps between the sounds

attune yourself to subtle changes in a speaker's tone, volume, and inflection

pack a lucky charm

attack a subject you are interested in

observe a florist at work

listen to the blood rush in your ears by cupping your hands over them

make up a new holiday for your favorite month

assign a day for taking care of pending papers in your home

hunt for hidden treasure

ask, "What would nature do?"

hold a glass to your mouth by sheer lung power

ask people to answer absurd hypothetical questions

have your hair done at home

make a list of all the books you have read

go through each book of your library

ask, "How can I help?"

give a flower to a stranger

get someone to play catch with you

focus a day on your sense of smell

find the lost remote control

fill the pet's food bowl

feel the grass between your toes

hard-boil eggs perfectly

ask someone what their current favorite
TV show is

experiment with color combinations

arrange your surroundings to encourage
harmony and enhance quality of life

dress up the cat

approach a problem by first figuring out
what won't work

draw on frosted glass

appreciate your hands

donate an old car to charity

appreciate an otherwise ordinary task

ask advice from the oldest person you
know

do your nail polish perfectly

apply for a scholarship

devise a treasure hunt for kids

answer the question: If you could do anything in this world right now, what would it be?

clean up the garage

do the training to answer a suicide hotline

clean a chandelier

allow your mind to relax

buy a red carnation and wear it to work

ask someone the time

build something out of toothpicks

create a list of values that you admire

ask questions in meetings and lectures

air out your home, or at least your bedroom

ask for help

get a foot massage

make a list of 10 questions for a project you are about to begin think about what you have learned from an animal

admire the wildflowers alongside the roadway

alternate reading a cookbook and a diet book

adjust a paper airplane to improve aerodynamics

look at funny pictures in your high school yearbook

add to your bird life list

allow yourself to be in the moment with its surprises

admire someone's knickknacks

adapt a novel for film

add a symbol to your signature (star, heart, flower, etc.)

act like wherever you are is the best place to be

say hello to a homeless person

absorb the sun and the feeling of being alive

learn reflexology

stroke someone's hair

fill a glass bowl with fresh fruit

eat outside on a nice day

brake for a rainbow

put a flower on someone's windshield

lengthen your steps when walking

go on a litter hunt

do the laundry on a sunny day and hang it out to dry

sell stuff on consignment

add an entry to a journal

compare notes and memories of a shared experience with the person you shared it with

open a door literally and see how it feels figuratively

spray cologne in dresser drawers

close your eyes and relax

check out the fire exits

practice the Zen art of one-pointedness, thinking of only one thing

ask not what computers can do, but what they should do

learn how to julienne, chiffonade, and dice

cook outdoors

get rid of leftovers

write a poem on the sidewalk with chalk

make gravy

breathe in for four counts, hold for four, breathe out for four, until you fall asleep

discard everything in a category all at once

create pictograms

take control of the portion size of your food

simplify your life

learn more about deep breathing

wait up for someone

prowl used bookstores, stalls, and marts

revel in time alone

write outdoors

play balloon volleyball

create dot patterns

shred cheese

garden with a child

sleep outdoors under the stars

while dining, alternate your knife and
    fork in each hand

beautify a beach

do a crossword puzzle or maze

take a nap in the shade of a tree

send your friends Christmas cards,
    whatever time of year

find a new use for a favorite old piece of
    clothing

shop at the local health food store

dry grapes to make raisins

notice lines and basic shapes

pretend that you are a leaf drifting along a quiet, lazy stream on a sunny day

start seeds indoors

ask to see the kitchen of a great restaurant

go to a petting zoo

instead of trying to figure it out, just notice it

create a list of all the toys you remember having as a child

learn to make pizza

notice patterns in your environment— stripes, zigzags, swirls, etc.

do a handstand in water

read *Good Night, Moon* to a child

sow a garden with heirloom seeds

rehabilitate an injury

come up with a plan B

buy lemonade from kids at a stand

write down all your blessings

force yourself to pay attention

walk a few steps behind people
    in conversation for subtle
    eavesdropping

shag softballs

treat yourself to a mud bath

pretend you're an archaeologist seeking
    the weirdest product in a big-box store

take an elderly neighbor to the
    supermarket when you go
    shopping

set up a spa in your bathroom

palm your eyes to calm and soothe
    yourself

learn how to say "This is delicious" in
    a new language 📱

snip the head of a drooping flower to
    place in a snifter of water

monogram your canvas tote

create balance in your mind

go grocery shopping in a very strange outfit

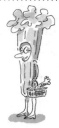

improve your mile run time

brainstorm

focus on the colors, flavors, textures, and temperatures of the parts of a meal

clean the lint off of Velcro attachments

fix a snack to share

breakfast outdoors

make a list of 10 songs that were important to you at different times

design your own logo or monogram

write a limerick

read about a new subject that interests you

watch a crab on the shore crawling backward in search of the ocean

notice individual raindrops

light a pink candle to increase loving
    feelings and enhance friendship

relive your fondest memory

build a fort with blankets

notice colors

make a list of 101 things to do with
    leftovers

count the petals of a flower

set all your clocks to exactly the right
    time

slow dance

paint a picket fence

darn any socks that have holes

notice the order in which you put on
    clothes

document the life of a garden

go for a ride

light a red candle for protection

play miniature golf

buy something completely indulgent at a bakery

find all the hidden cat toys

visualize walking through peaceful places

power-wash the house and the lawn furniture

treat a friend to a meal

drink milk from the container

learn math tricks

make today's to-do list

mingle with friends or strangers

envision every muscle getting stronger

look for friendly faces

acquire fun facts from books

install a password protector on all your computers 📱

go snowshoeing

count all the trees you can see from where you are

donate five things you don't need

make a list as long as your arm of things
   to be happy about

mull cider

create a landscape painting of your town

make finger sandwiches

take a genius or Mensa test

cleanse your internal organs through
   yoga twists

crumple up your to-do list

whistle

start a discussion about a special interest

freeze some snowballs

plan a gourmet meal

catch something important before it
   gets away

keep a list of all the books you read,
   along with your favorite passages

practice tai chi or martial arts moves

design a gourmet chef's kitchen

restart your oldest hobby

work on a journal article

cut down or choose a Christmas tree

try to go to sleep by listening intently and trying to identify every sound or noise

allow thoughts and ideas to rise from your creative depths

take your papers to be shredded

gather up new ideas and run with them

make butter cookies

finish a craft project

cram one more thing into the garbage can

find an oasis

train the dog to catch a Frisbee

enjoy the morning sun

count at least five blessings of the day

draw a paper bag

notice what light does to objects at different times of the day

decorate a pair of cheap canvas sneakers with permanent markers

inhale mouth-watering aromas from nearby restaurants

culture yogurt at home

clip the nail that is bothering you

occupy a blanket fort

do math longhand

take a leap of faith

decode the psychological messages that accompany objects

listen to that hunch

undertake a new challenge

read with a pencil in your hand

cherish the memory of someone

serve meals to the homeless

add special touches to your home

press flowers or fall leaves in books

join a flag football team

eat, drink, and be merry

create an Etch-A-Sketch masterpiece

choose a moment to commit to your
memory bank

make unusual lists—a party's memorable
moments, celebrities you saw in
public places, etc.

divide your books into daily reading
portions

rattle off trivia

finish your errands during lunch hour

play horseshoes

balance your chakras

use a seesaw in a park

bring order to chaos at work

identify 10 strengths you are proud of

disassemble things and study them from
different perspectives

get "lost" in a forest

break the habit of waiting—just do stuff

list 10 things other than keys that can be carried on a key chain

let your imagination soar

create pointillism pictures

look at everything and everybody around you as though you're seeing them for the first time

change where pictures are displayed

shower praise on someone

embrace the ordinary

gather a bunch of flowers

dig up a couch potato and get them to go on a walk with you

put classical music on a sleep timer

take pictures of items you are getting rid of so you have a visual memento of them

visit a monument

create a lair

parrot sentences in a foreign phrase book

light a white candle to promote peace
and spirituality

license your dog

watch the moon

build and paint a bird feeder

try a mantra

spread a little joy

make your guest room into a destination
for mini-retreats

lighten your schedule

have a long, thoughtful conversation

get rid of every item of clothing that
doesn't look good on you

learn to make jewelry

discuss what cloud shapes look like

do a handstand against a tree
or wall

learn your state's history, what its name means, etc.

find a new recipe to try

combine information from separate sources to reach a new conclusion

dress like your favorite person

figure out how to use *Roget's Thesaurus*

amble with a sketchbook or camera

make ice cream soup

oil and break in a baseball glove

leave everything a little better than you found it

get a flu shot

ask advice from a youngster

plant an edible garden

find the key that fits the lock

make croutons

do a blind taste test on tap water, bottled water, and rainwater

prune any deadwood from shrubs

make a keepsake box

order delivery from a nearby restaurant

pick up five pieces of litter and then congratulate yourself

spruce up the room by moving items around or tidying

watch batting practice

browse the farmers market

cultivate compassion for others

teach someone to cook your favorite dish

speak to someone you have never spoken to before

conceive a wonderful new plan for next weekend

put a flower on someone's pillow

plant radishes

go to a parking lot carnival

do a "kid thing" that you never did before

eat after brushing your teeth

go on a knowledge adventure by
reading about something you know
absolutely nothing about

plan an evening of entertaining at home

do the laundry

download an app to tune a musical
instrument 🔲

get everything together to go
tobogganing

deseed a watermelon

sing

banish useless thoughts

be still and completely open and
receptive to whatever comes into
your field of awareness

jump a wide puddle

cook your next meal as if
it is rare and expensive

time how long you can hold your breath

clip fascinating articles

breathe at a stoplight

draw a fantasy city

go for a swim and hold your breath underwater

notice sunlight illuminating the redness of a tomato

bathe by candlelight

perform an act of goodness or kindness

watch two clouds and "race" them

jump on the bed

make a journal of childhood memories

fetch the paper

take a new driving route

show affection

decide to overcome a challenge in your life

prowl the shops

repair ripped jeans

organize shoes and handbags

return to a creative outlet you had earlier in your life

set aside some money to spend at a later date

watch planes land

count cows along the roadside

marinate an idea

wash dishes by hand

paint eggs for an Easter egg hunt

tell ghost stories and toast marshmallows

leap like a kangaroo

tell time by the sun

learn a breathing exercise to help you doze off at night

eat Doritos or Oreos without guilt

do cross-training

reach the word count required for a paper

glance at the sky as you head home from work

enjoy communal happiness, feeling part of the crowd

reexamine your priorities

transform pots, pans, and wooden spoons into a drum set

test-drive a car

crack open a bottle of red wine and allow it to breathe

pat the cat

skip as you walk

help find homes for stray pets

find a cause to donate time to

clean to calm your inner chaos

watch butter melt on toast

make a homemade milkshake

shift the tone of a gripe session with humor

replace blown light bulbs

take a test for something you have not trained in, like selling real estate

set a timer for 20 minutes and get
work done

look for flying saucers

allot part of your lunch hour to
movement like walking, yoga,
or light aerobics

pause and expand your awareness to the
edges of your visual field

collect all your canvas shopping bags to
use instead of plastic ones

clean paintbrushes

create fractal art

get rid of instruction manuals for stuff
you no longer own

consult the *I Ching*

dry herbs

finish unfinished business, whether
large or small

pick a new thought and focus all your
energy on it

celebrate a moment in life that you'd otherwise deem ordinary

read a dictionary page

replace a zipper pull with a ribbon

write a letter to yourself

roller-skate or rollerblade

watch a cook prepare a meal

open an old box of keepsakes or photographs

do something nice for someone

put away your art or crafting supplies

build a fort for a pet or a child

meditate for five minutes

clean out the bird cage

sweep under the rug

make an English breakfast

deter a friend from making a mistake

ask a local where you can find something beautiful in the area

research a historical event

pick up a baguette for dinner

rearrange your kitchen so everything
   needed is within reach

invent a new dance

try tae bo

make a homemade beanbag

whisk whipping cream

go forest bathing

lay out clothes for the morning

eat a fancy lunch out alone

practice yoga

create a household bulletin board

shred and recycle office papers

bounce a ball off a wall where the noise
   won't bother anyone

play relaxing music

make a key chain

build mountains with mashed potatoes,
   adding gravy lava

talk to someone you see every day but do not know

skate backward

pretend you are a tightrope walker

convince your partner to do something spontaneous with you

crosshatch a drawing

align pictures in a room by the tops of their frames

make the first move

crack a nut

figure out the closest place you can go for a weekend getaway

locate your passport and check the expiration date

implement space-saving ideas

explore a hidden world under a log

learn to love weeding

discover a new trail

dance with just your upper body

complete a difficult task

breathe deeply

change your handbag or wallet

spring-clean one room

wash the microfiber cloths and dustcloths

research organizations to donate to

make a hiking stick

grow tomatoes

have a heart-to-heart

examine your morning routine and
shake it up

find a mistake in a dictionary

bask on a rock in the sun

learn how to identify animal tracks

listen to a famous aria, such as one from
Carmen

inspect the art on a dollar bill

throw a come-as-you-are party

make candles

think of interesting new questions to ask
friends and partners

re-cover a piece of furniture

teach a cat to fetch

look at everyday objects under
a magnifying glass

listen to the classical soundtracks from
Looney Tunes cartoons

turn your face to the sun, wherever you
are

make a cold soup

bring nature inside

share a crossword puzzle

count fireflies

set a goal to score a goal in any sport

liberate someone from a typically
gender-based task

read the labels and tags on your clothes

unlock the door for someone

put your jacket around someone on
a chilly evening

double-check your spelling before
sending an email

locate the North Star

perfect your expertise at a pub game—
darts, billiards, trivia, etc.

set your hair in curlers

participate in a race or competition

beautify your yard, garden, or
neighborhood

put all your important papers in the
same envelope

organize a favorite collection

let someone go ahead of you in line

cover a bulletin board with positive
affirmations and photos

notice happy sounds around you

name your future boat

challenge something you know

make sure gloves are in the car

decorate the envelope of the next letter
    you send

bob for apples

start a conversation

rub prayer beads

create a home office

splurge on fresh flowers

plan a dinner party

resist doing anything

start a journal of who you are and how
    you feel

repot plants

design a flag

clean for five minutes

leave a quarter where a child can find it

be aware of the signs around you

hang a sign in a park calling people's
    attention to something special

paint a landscape

go out to dinner

notice the fashions worn by everyone in a public place

give yourself a treat and take the time to really enjoy it

go for a moonlit hike

fill out college applications

construct an elaborate but realistic fantasy

do an art project using three different media or techniques

do squat thrusts

go to a paint-your-own-ceramics studio

count sheep

do a life inventory

practice the ability to levitate

decide to keep dinner simple and prepare it in under 30 minutes

dry flowers

dance in the dark

create a nom de guerre for yourself

make a handheld fan

develop extraordinary powers of
observation

take a fitness test

come up with an impressive piece of
writing

find your niche

mountain-bike

climb a rope

pass on your wisdom to someone

begin a meal by giving thanks, even
silently

pick up and feel the produce at the
farmers market

become a Big Brother or Big Sister

geocache on a hike

bake a crock of beans

do triceps dips on a chair

go to a nursing home and spend time
    with someone who has no visitors

allocate resting places for your glasses,
    keys, wallet, and slippers so you can
    always find them

write lyrics to a passionate love song

rub and press reflexology points on your
    hands and feet

whip up a casserole

turn tidying the house into a game

watch your clothes dryer's spin cycle

unpack clothes from the dry cleaner

wait for the exact moment the first star
    appears in the night sky

leave time to read before falling asleep

vacuum the couch

compose music

try something new on the menu

pet your pet

train for a triathlon

satisfy an itch, literally or figuratively

trace a love message in the sand

juggle dinner rolls

thank the person who sells tickets

splash in the puddles

test the smoke detectors

attach a love note to your partner's
computer screen

sew or construct a Halloween costume

identify a self-defeating behavior and
create steps to change

put a flower in your hair

freeze fruit to eat frozen or
put in smoothies

**study everything except the
art in a museum**

gather all the mystery cords
in your home and throw
them away

fry up some bacon

open a dictionary and read about the first word you see

arm-wrestle

create a hand-drawn typeface

arrange something—pencils, shirts in your closet, etc.—by color

schedule a time to get your fishing license

share food with others

go on a juice fast

look for flickers of individuality within the routine of the everyday

cook yourself a good breakfast

find the joy in wondering about the toilet paper roll or that coffee cup lid

get earwax removed by a professional

feel the earth beneath your feet

play hide-and-seek

check out someone else's doodles

mend clothing

teach yourself to do something new
without watching the clock

do squat exercises using a chair

teach someone to ride a bike

check something off your bucket list

take up interval training

learn all the bones in the body

give a stray cat some water or milk

finish reading a half-read book

sweep the front walk

eat alone in public

pin up your hair

stop, pick up a found object, and
determine whether it is interesting

bring fresh flowers to work

punch the pillow

stare out at calm water

calculate the possible consequences of
an action

learn to listen, not just to hear

be on time

perform a selfless act

adapt to the pace of nature around you

make up your own lyrics to an
   existing song

plant corn in the backyard

**spend the first 10 minutes of
the day outside**

remember to drink eight glasses of
   water a day

sit on a pier and watch the happenings

put on boots and tramp through wet
   fields and woods

share your seat or bench

learn the aviation alphabet from alpha
   to zulu

seek a guru

help a child use a dictionary

see what flowers are growing in your
   local park

explore other offices in a building you are in

catch a falling leaf to make a wish come true or for a day of good luck

run in the rain

create music using kitchen objects

learn how to forecast the weather with a pinecone

replace a doorsill

hide delightful things for others to discover

renew your license plate registration

explore different career or life paths

have a good cry

support an independent local business

find a mentor

go kayaking

remove a roadblock

gently jostle for space on a crowded train

reflect on the day that is in the process of becoming yesterday

write a letter to your descendants

make a birdhouse out of a gourd

jump rope to a childhood rhyme

polish your shoes

redecorate your office

build a fence out of snow

see things from a bird's point of view

rearrange a room

walk wherever you like and see what happens

read to someone

kiss and make up

flip through an old diary

set five goals for the year

create a glossary for the subject you know best

remind someone to do something

jump on a trampoline

watch a cat stalking a bird

do freelance work

try a love potion

return books to the library

make your desk setup ergonomically correct

try sketch-noting, a method of note-taking that relies on thumbnail drawings

figure out how to turn your avocation into your vocation

try falling asleep with one eye open

put up storage shelves

dog-walk for a neighbor

read a cookbook

lift weights

clean out the attic, basement, or garage

transplant cuttings to the garden

prep the lawn mower

tie-dye a T-shirt

pore over a newspaper

change out aerosols for non-aerosols

plan an adventurous expedition

vary the order in which you do your
    morning routine

make a friendship bracelet

talk back to self-doubt

watch the mist lift

look at clothing fibers through a
    microscope

identify an actor to play you in your
    life story

pick your biographer

storyboard an idea

paint a wall a bright color

remember a forgotten memory

ask open-ended questions

notice something you've never noticed
    before

shake the rugs outside

peruse library books for ideas

listen to old rafters, creaky doors, and loose floorboards

train yourself to nap for 10 minutes

read a how-to book

meditate on a fish tank

get rid of gifts you have saved if you do not use or like them

massage your feet before bed

play tiddlywinks

identify the source of the sounds in your office

choose an issue you're struggling with and work with it

join a community garden

analyze your dreams

create an entire coloring book

mix juices to make a new flavor

choose a meaningful project

volunteer at a recreation program

make something out of an empty box

take the long way home

make homemade ice cream

solve a mystery

make a food dish from scratch using only
the ingredients you have at hand

pretend to be a tourist

listen for power lines humming

play with Bubble Wrap

let a dog walk you for a change

plant a kiss on someone's palm and close
it up for later use

learn about a friend's special interest
or talent

look at trinkets in a local shop

list all the ice cream flavors you have ever
tried

jump rope double Dutch style

learn a new job skill

cannonball into a deep pool

go to a museum gift shop

get your driver's license verified or
renewed

create a packing list for a day at school
or work

drive to the country and stop at all the
farm stands

jot down one-liners

decide what to wear tomorrow

join the neighborhood association

clean your hairbrush and comb

invite a friend to camp in the backyard or
on the porch

clean the countertops

indulge in a guilty pleasure

check the dates on everything in the
refrigerator and cupboards

identify the current phase of the moon

attend an event at your local church,
synagogue, or temple

identify a bird you've never seen before

water your garden

join an investment club

hit the golf course

watch shadows dapple the floor

hide a freckle

play hopscotch

hang up or put away all clothes that are
lying around

walk barefoot in the park

make a flowchart

donate the vegetables from your garden
to the local soup kitchen

map a new route home from work

pop on a pair of sunglasses so you can
people-watch in secret

grow a squash or pumpkin

shred a guitar

search a social situation for a poignant
moment

do 30 abdominal crunches

give your pet a mini spa treatment

browse new car lots

give the gift of undivided attention

pile all the clothes you own on a bed and
keep only what brings you joy

get some people time

take Sunday papers to the park

get ready for tryouts

dry a gourd

get off the hamster wheel you created
for yourself

learn to lay a fire

sit in the car and listen to the radio
without going anywhere

sketch a favorite scene with undivided
attention

get all the lumps out of the gravy

be aware of the space between your
thoughts

garden in the winter

hula-hoop

look for equipment and supplies for hobbies that you no longer pursue and part with them

farm your own land

put an article of clothing on inside out

confess your sins in total seclusion

fold a paper fan

cover scratches on furniture

find something symmetrical

eat cereal for dinner

find out the book value of your car

design your dream roller coaster

explore an art store

jaywalk at the mall

make a flint tool

take a nap outside

exercise at lunch

inhale helium from a balloon to speak in a silly voice

start a contagious yawn

rebuild an engine

plan a detoxification treatment

look up mind-mapping and then try mind-mapping a tough decision 📱

just *be*

keep a gratitude journal

alphabetize CDs, DVDs, or tapes

design a dress

learn through practice

work on a creative project

soak dishes or pans before trying to clean them

try to facilitate greater understanding between people at work

make pesto

create a gel hairstyle

alphabetize and replace expired items in the spice rack

have a friend over

tire out the children

draw a smiley face on the closest available surface

find a mantra

contribute to a local cause

take your morning coffee break with a compassionate coworker

peer out windows late at night, marveling at the muted dusting of stars against a blue velvet sky

finish a chore

pawn off an unwanted errand

make a miniature flower arrangement

support a friend

go on a walk and feel gratitude for nature

focus completely on each step of a particular task

attempt the impossible

admit you were wrong

find an intriguing item in an antique store and seek out its history

observe people on a commuter train

enjoy the last bite of chocolate

recapture a favorite childhood activity

make a finger ring out of a dollar bill

pick a new name

read while taking a bath

make an Easter egg tree

decorate a gift box

ask a librarian what his or her favorite book is

examine your furniture and make a list of touch-ups you can do yourself

give honest feedback

examine a prejudice

jog a mile

fit every last thing in the dishwasher

eat the chip or cookie crumbs

kick your favorite exercise routine up a notch

eat at an odd site

draw what each season means to you

frame an inspirational print and put it where you will see it often

enjoy a period of rest

drive a mower

unpack the groceries while listening to pop music

make decorated storage containers for the kitchen

draw an object you see without lifting the pencil off the page

select categories and make lists of all the things you can think of for each

paint a house

navigate through a dimly lit house

notice the contours of a cat or dog's body

do crosswords in ink

go for a midnight picnic

correct your posture

pick a part of your life to downsize and
get started

get a facial

donate books to a school or public library

find the ingredients you need

make a family yearbook

watch as dusk falls

fill all the reusable water bottles and put
them in the fridge

**pat yourself on the back for
whatever you did today**

donate a jug of fruit salad to
a senior center

paint and re-caulk the storm
windows

do yoga or stretches before bed

do things that are normally outside of
your routine

tour the town at night

concentrate on every bite of food

zest a lemon

do all the quizzes in a spelling book

scale down your purse size

dispose of old paint cans and other
maintenance items no longer used
or needed

preheat the oven or grill

write a letter and include a sweet story

make meatloaf

create a fresh flower arrangement

put anything that catches your eye into
your sketchbook

watch a cat sleep

bury the hatchet with an old friend

make popovers

build a dollhouse

find a perfectly ripe avocado at the store

discover something new about
something familiar

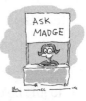

**offer counsel to those who
seek it**

design the perfect tree house
for your favorite tree

measure the snow

delight in the simple joy of a long walk

credit your sources of inspiration

decorate with feng shui

learn to identify crystals

declare a thumb war

sit somewhere with a great view and
a great friend

make a family tree diagram

traverse an old stone bridge

dare to do something you're anxious
about doing

keep up with a pen pal

dance the mambo

fix a misunderstanding between friends

tea-dye fabric

cut your pet's nails

become alert to unfamiliar vocabulary
that you hear or read and look it
up later

cut out junk thoughts

run laps

create the illusion of sunlight with
a candle and a halogen lamp

tease your cat with a laser pointer

create art with sidewalk chalk

aerate soil

craft a replica artifact

drive, breathe, and reflect in silence

count your change

sail a leaf boat

do a difficult yoga pose

change the linens on the bed

catch snowflakes

make a family schedule

come up with a positive phrase

cook dinner in the fireplace

read a chapter in a book

clean out kitchen cupboards

put colored light bulbs in your lamps

plan an eat-with-your-hands dinner party

euphemize what you say

go to a local spa for a treatment

design handbags

listen to old 45s on a turntable

unpack

investigate the origin of a word

propagate bulbs

invent a game

explore a new place on foot

line closet shelves with scented paper

write down all the weird things you wonder about

figure out the six ways a batter can get on base without a hit

walk a dog for a sick neighbor

create a flip-book with index cards

install wickets for croquet or baskets for disc golf

treat yourself to a massage

decorate for the next holiday

take an early or late lunch and work without interruption when everyone else is at lunch

set up a café for dinner

enjoy getting your hands dirty

assemble a LEGO village

build time into your schedule for brainstorming ideas

put the first footprints in new-fallen snow

dowse for water

prepare an emergency or "go" bag

cook with a kid

hit tennis balls against a backboard

look for earthworms

buff the car

make a list of clothes you need for the next season

trace over something you want to learn to draw

sign up for a course at the local or community college

adjust your posture

read a humorously inappropriate meaning into a sign you see

train your cat or dog to walk a figure eight

get to know the geology of your area

practice being a flaneur

have a free throw–shooting contest

nap outdoors

focus on something small on a wall for as
long as you can

season a cast-iron pan

fix a rift in your family

get warm by a fire

unsubscribe from all email
advertisements 📱

decorate a pair of jeans

go for a swim

count the number of birds you see in five
minutes

play tic-tac-toe on the paper tablecloth
where you are eating

write your life story

become absorbed with the mystery of the
environment

volunteer as a docent

scent your home without candles

use your fireplace

practice doing a great impression of a celebrity

throw out ingredients that do not agree with you

learn survival skills

tell a joke

pile leaves into huge heaps and jump in

study a painting

put on perfume

get rid of "just in case" storage boxes

eat a meal with chopsticks

spend time hibernating

taste a dish while you're cooking

make a fairy garden

grow your own vegetables and herbs

put extra cherries on your sundae

bargain at a bazaar

smell the freshness of a rain shower

paste quotes, dreams, ticket stubs, and pictures into a journal sharpen the kitchen knives

eat something as you shop and pay for it at the checkout

send a fan letter

play pool

seek out behind-the-scenes sites

become an urban explorer

memorize something word for word

seek awe in the heavens—the moon through a telescope, a star shooting through the sky

search for caves in the woods

spread some kindness

do tomorrow's homework

bring two brown-bag lunches to a friend's house

create a five-year plan

recalibrate your bicycle

watch the horizon glow

play cards

complete a half-finished DIY project

make your Christmas wish list

make lemons into lemonade

play Who am I?

make soup from ingredients you have in
the kitchen right now

bury or hide a treasure for someone and
make a map for it

put something in your shoe so you don't
forget it when you leave

make a pomander

put something in its proper place

oil things that don't move smoothly

figure out how to squeeze oranges and
then use all the other parts

pull a really fun all-nighter

see how you'd look with a mole above
your lip like Marilyn Monroe

explore back roads and quiet lanes

practice for team tryouts

pretend you are a superhero

consolidate and piggyback errands

play the spoons

massage someone's scalp

perform a service that makes a difference in your community

chew consciously

incubate a creative project

go on a full-moon hike

create smiley faces out of your fruit at breakfast

do the hokey pokey and shake it all about

organize school supplies

open a book to any page and let a paragraph or line inspire you

wander by bicycle

close your eyes and listen to the sounds of nature and people around you

clip comics you love

check out someone else's bookcases

gather signatures for a petition

offer to give your partner a neck or back
rub

offer a compliment to a stressed-out
associate

move some paintings around

mend a fishing net

give thanks

grow one tall sunflower in the front yard

draw your family flag

fill a sketchbook with ideas

sign up for a cooking lesson

set short-term and long-term goals

start a conga line while waiting for the
bus or train

drive quietly and notice your emotions

plan a cookout

learn to hacky sack

start journaling about your five senses

do a crossword puzzle as fast as you can

design a desk

learn memory techniques

practice cloud bursting, assigning each
    cloud a worry and watching it drift
    away

master a magic trick

look up instead of down

let silence empower you

light a candle for someone you are
    concerned about

imitate a birdsong

do push-ups

help someone in need

watch waves crashing

create a finger-paint masterpiece

disguise or hide the power cords

have an astrologer cast your chart

cover someone's eyes and lead them to
    a lovely surprise

hang out happily

bring orange slices for your sports team

think up a new response to someone who has just sneezed

dance down a supermarket aisle

give away pots, pans, and dishes you never use

write a how-to book on your subject of expertise

get up and walk outside

watch a cat on catnip

make a difference in the life of someone you care about

do something generous

get the ironing done

build a firepit outside

go to a hands-on museum

visit a formal garden

get out of a tight spot

talk to your plants

get an hour's work done before
anyone gets up

finish the laundry for someone

play a kazoo

be a neighborhood detective

find new purpose in old porch furniture

feed your pet a treat

make the final payment on something

examine the knots in the wood of the
floor

follow a child's movements

get a free makeover at a cosmetic counter

find the highest and lowest points in your
current emotional state

explore a city at a leisurely browser's
pace

feel the direction of the wind with the
fine hairs on your skin

discover a new secret hiding place

empty the pencil sharpener

dust the light fixtures

change your hairstyle

drive around in search of a particular type of architecture, like an old barn

volunteer on a farm

dig out a treasured family recipe to cook

collect all the unused clothes hangers in one place

listen to night sounds

satisfy all five senses

come up with a personal name for a piece of furniture

watch clouds change shape

look up how to stop a snore

rearrange family pictures

find a lost toy

feed ducks at a nearby pond

develop your own philosophy

sign up for a fun or impractical course

create a capsule wardrobe

find your own philosophy of living

take a tour of a local church

look for dust bunnies wherever you are

create an engraving

develop a secret formula

compose a concert using songs you love

blow out your hair

commit to finishing a drawing, no matter how bad you think it is

open up all your senses

pray for the welfare of a friend or family member

assemble a piece of furniture

camp out in the backyard

bounce bits of trivia off someone

practice perspective drawing

balance a spinning basketball

re-create your favorite restaurant meal at home

file important papers in
 permanent storage

shadow a mentor

appreciate the flora of the season

donate dictionaries to a school

combine two or more senses in
 unexpected ways, like listening to a
 piece of music while smelling freshly
 baked cookies

volunteer with a literacy program

clear and organize your desk

paint a fresco

clear the table after a meal

create a filing system that works

notice the color and texture of snow

create a daily diary in your pet's voice

go for a long walk with the wind

think of book recommendations for your
 favorite TV characters

finish one thing you have been putting off

go dancing

chronicle your daily walk

scrub a really dirty pot

open yourself up to a heightened state of awareness

change what you can change and stop worrying about the rest

watch dust in the sun

devise seven workouts you can rotate that do not involve a gym

clarify butter

change a "no" to a "yes"

bring plants back from the brink of death

challenge yourself to focus on one thing at a time, slow down, and do less

light candles

celebrate the holidays of all the religions

decide how to change a bad habit you have

taste test two new kinds of cheese

put notebooks in every room of the house for jotting down thoughts

catch up on your reading

cobble together a plan for a project

care for children

verbalize nouns

campaign to save the manatees

fix a hem

call a parent just to say hi

have seconds

build an igloo

revive a forgotten hobby

brush your teeth mindfully

consider what you'd write on a billboard

browse a nearby shop

make breakfast for dinner

make a diagram of how something makes
  you feel

start composting

bring in positive energy through the top
  of your head

peel an orange in one shot

bring a coloring book and crayons for
  your wait

sort shopping bags by size

become expert at making fires both in
  the fireplace and at a campsite

sing with kids in the car

become an expert sauce chef

do jumping jacks

be an anonymous donor

try to read a cat's mind

eat dessert before dinner

be alert to a stranger who might actually
  inspire you

stock a bunker in case of emergency

attempt to describe beautiful places through art, music, or writing

spend 10 minutes looking out the window you forget about most

at the end of the day, note five things you did for others

play gin rummy

ask your mother or father to tell you a story

take cuttings of plants

learn to draw

twirl a baton

clean out junk drawers

do a craft with kids

curl your hair

change the kitty litter

kneel down to pet a dog or cat

pick a name for a new pet

deep-clean contact lenses

create a fantasy deli spread

untie your shoes

make an art journal out of an old dictionary

learn calculus

ask a good question

trim the hedges

remember to do your sit-ups

play baseball

make a daisy chain

consider who you might have been in a former life

put on a tiny wash-off tattoo

inhale negative karma, difficulties, and conflicting emotions, then exhale them as happiness and joy

learn the art of wire wrapping

adjust the thermostat

help a child prepare for a spelling bee

pit an avocado

explore the earth

stretch out in an empty bathtub
and read

catch a dream and interpret it

hang new wind chimes

use a lint roller on furniture

empty your handbag and remove
unneeded stuff

train a cat to walk on a leash

sit still like a frog on a lily pad—at ease,
but present and alert

throw away love letters from someone
who broke your heart

go exploring off the beaten path

tell someone how you really feel

play with your food

take something downstairs

study the biography of someone you
admire

endow a scholarship

stop to listen to the storm

bang on kitchen pots

list every gift you remember
    receiving

spin a globe, put your finger on a spot,
    and plan a fantasy trip

dream with your eyes wide open

spend an hour in a coffee shop or mall
    and then write about it

make frozen juice pops

spend a day in bed writing your memoir

put winter clothes in storage

practice a few minutes of "toning": singing
    or chanting elongated vowels

look at an object until you see something
    new

make a cucumber, radish, or watercress
    sandwich

depict a great scene in words

take a cold shower

forgive yourself for that mistake you
    keep thinking about

wash delicates in the sink

play basketball on a vacant outdoor court at dusk

cook a fancy breakfast on Saturday morning

put a dollar into a piggy bank

watch a video on how to do decorative finishes on furniture 📱

get rid of cosmetic samples you've gotten from stores

go on a field trip

scratch pets behind the ears or under the chin

do the hard thing, not the easy thing

narrate what you are cooking as if you were on the Food Network

pay attention to strange shapes

kick a beach or soccer ball

pack a healthy lunch

march in place

observe a craftsperson working

decode a message written in Morse code

make up a new game

test all your pens

go to a favorite outdoor spot early in the morning and watch the sun come up

powder your nose

punch a punching bag

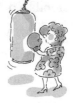

have a deep conversation with a sibling

learn shorthand

find a long-lost something

rank the holidays you celebrate from favorite to least favorite

hold a garage sale

turn about-face

create a family trivia game

rummage for finds at a flea market

have your hair blown out at a salon

come up with a new signature

go through an old family album

gather fall leaves for an indoor
    decoration

make a crown of flowers

touch trees

stitch and bitch

focus a day on sight

visit a loved one's grave

fill the ice cube trays

do bookbinding repairs

concoct your own breakfast juice
    combination

experiment with color

swat an insect

write a horoscope for someone you care
    about

find a no-knead recipe for homemade
    bread

watch a candle flicker

correct a mistake

look for chimneys

help another over a rough spot in the
   road of life

do something fun

acknowledge small but precious bonding
   moments with a stranger

build a collage file

practice child's pose

dress up for no reason

pump up all the sports balls

work off your meal

make confetti

hunt for ambient sounds, feelings,
   patterns, shapes, and colors

donate an art box to a needy child

clean fur out of the cat bed

do your hair in braids

fill a bucket with autumn flowers

visualize what you want to most change
   about yourself

devise a recipe for a bake-off

do five things that you are afraid to do

clean up after yourself

pick one thing while on a walk, pause, and take time to really attend to it

make a personalized map of the town you live in

adjust your bicycle

start a compost pile

stock the fridge

listen to kids at play

return everything you have borrowed

plan a camping trip

drink lots of water

keep a dream diary

flirt

design a coffee table to be used as a footrest

wander around an old church

work on a car

remove calluses with a pumice stone

try to draw something you see each day

convert a wild tangle into a garden

remove your makeup

split your big project into smaller,
    easy-to-achieve tasks

finish a book

snoop around like Nancy Drew

draw variations on the theme of good,
    better, best

enjoy the fresh, clear quietness of
    a country morning

untangle an impossible knot

ask, "How can I be of service?"

draw a great political cartoon

work outdoors

decorate a flowerpot

drum a rhythm

clean a bathtub

count railroad cars as they pass

buy a painting from an up-and-coming
artist

get together with old friends

create a dish that is different from the
usual season specialties

dance the samba

do a core strength workout

make a confession

feed an abandoned baby bird

take a city dog for a walk in the
country

watch the grass grow

find the funny side of a situation

try a little bit of everything at a buffet

feel the corners of your mouth
curling up

do an unexpected favor for your boss

soak your feet in hot water for 20
minutes

figure out how to fold a fitted sheet

do a loving-kindness meditation for
  yourself and others

build something amazing with someone

reevaluate and edit your wardrobe

ask questions before sleeping, then
  dream the answers

drive on a new highway

ask for attention or a hug

tackle one nagging task

arrange a cheese plate

do Neurobic brain exercises

alternate between a sitting meditation
  and a mindful walk

turn on the porch light for someone
  returning home later

allow your mind to become empty

find hidden compartments in things you
  already own

admire someone's collection of
  knickknacks

walk backward somewhere

add a plant to a room

press a hot spoon on a bug bite

arrange to have a microchip implanted in your pet

walk out your door and hike at least five miles

relish the ecstatic experience of fresh air and wind in your face

study ikebana, the art of Japanese flower arranging

allow a smile to travel within you and rest in your abdomen, radiating warmth and joy

look over a test and catch a mistake

admire a great sample of your handwriting

shadowbox

make a collage of your baby pictures

act on a hunch

sleep in another part of the house

celebrate your own creativity

serve dinner with artistry

choose an outfit with your eyes closed

randomly choose which restaurant
to go to

open any book in a bookstore and find
a moral lesson

offer something you are done with to
another

become especially well-read in
something

smell something new

change waiting time to thinking time

run along the water's edge

play stickball

choose an exotic fruit at the grocery store

stay by a river or waterfall for a long
period of time

pluck a banjo

cut the grass

stay to help clean up after an event or
    meeting

read a book you were supposed to read in
    high school or college

make beautiful and surprising
    interruptions in your life by talking
    to strangers

clean out file cabinets

wander through a warehouse store

pick up an instrument and practice

wash the car windows on the inside

invent a font

turn your desk so you can see out
    the window

eat a communal silent meal

throw a boomerang

create your own chili recipe

think of a sound that reminds you
    of childhood and reminisce

lose your thoughts in the sound
    of the wind

create a diorama with a peephole in
   one end

sit in a spot and imagine the
   pictures you could take

teach a cat to sit and stay

make a collage of mementos
   of special events

clip out a *New Yorker* cartoon

unjam a drawer

learn to do self-hypnosis

set a clock

freshen the blankets with lavender spray

read the footnotes

research yurts to vacation in

put your house in order room by room

walk a mile in someone else's shoes

plan the family reunion

smile at your reflection

perfect your bubble-blowing technique

collect ideas

participate in a fun run

have a day of complete relaxation

find a hideout

organize a family photograph

people-watch from a park bench

name your car

watch the sunrise and the neighborhood wake up

make sure every room of your home is multicolored

look at an infinite horizon with attention and focus

leave a note for an event's host describing what made the party great

allow gratitude to expand throughout your being

hang a planter

slow-cook a meal

take yourself out to brunch

string beads

give yourself a pep talk

time how long the sun is out before
a cloud obscures it

fill out all the forms necessary for a new
school, job, or project

select new eyeglasses

do an anonymous good deed

make a basketball and hoop out of paper,
then play the game

discover laziness and allow yourself to
delight in it

make a collage from whatever you can
find in the room you're in

resolve to find happiness today

take a caffeine nap, drinking caffeine and
then napping 20 minutes later

dance in front of a mirror

go to a comedy club

compile a current list of all birthdays and
special anniversaries

paint a dream

climb a ladder

examine the color of coffee

begin a journal in a blank book

go for a listening walk

choose a part of your personality you can
improve upon

say a centering prayer

bake a cake or batch of cookies and eat as
much as you want

take your dog to an agility training class

adopt a new belief

delve into poetry

disguise cottage cheese in a recipe

pay yourself a compliment

nap on the beach

practice downward dog and stay there for
five breaths

observe bees pollinating flowers

dash off a postcard

prepare your questions for a tarot card reading

draw treasure maps

cut sandwiches into different geometric shapes

skip rope

console a crying baby

look for and document minor flaws around you

paint drawer handles different colors

shoot hoops

put a condiment smile on someone's sandwich or burger

pray for a political figure you disagree with

go on a day's adventure

make Kool-Aid

make a Christmas wreath

read a field guide

create a detective character

scrape snow and ice off the car

do your own happy dance

help clean a polluted beach

open a book to a page, point, and use the
    word or phrase to launch a project

craft paper flowers

close your eyes and *listen*

patch clothes

identify a bird by its chirp

do a cobweb painting

move the furniture around

capture and document thoughts,
    sentiments, observations,
    ruminations, and reflections

check out an ethnic grocery store

drive through farm country during
    a summer sunset

mix two salad dressing recipes to create
    a new one

pick fresh flowers for your house

throw garbage across the room
and try to make the wastebasket

turn out the lights

settle into the present moment

collect loose change in a jar

draw with pastels

put chargers in strategic places around
the house

mull over a personal matter

use a bath bomb and immerse yourself in
the soapy bathwater

turn one small activity into a meditative
ritual

practice *tonglen*, breathing in the
suffering of the world and breathing
out peace and happiness

write a great eulogy

interview someone

watch a butterfly sunning itself on a
flower

play Animal, vegetable, or mineral?

do something frivolous

make a Christmas tree ornament

learn how to do a proper table setting

deliver compassion

build a coatrack

practice walking a very thin line

retry a food you don't like

backpack through a local natural wonder

window-shop

bathe a pet

dust, then vacuum

plump the doggy bed

listen and look for bugs in the woods

do self-ethnography, documenting your
own life and culture

hide secret notes all over the house

jump off the bandwagon

ship a package

get rid of clothes that you have
   downgraded to loungewear

notice five things in your vicinity that
   have changed recently

shave your legs

discover that the less you say, the more
   you hear

**balance something on
   your head**

prebake a piecrust

join a bowling league

create an emergency kit

design new packaging for something
   that's currently poorly packaged

choose a color that you like and look for
   it everywhere

write up a list of life goals

volunteer at a hospital

trudge up a hill

take the dog for a swim

tell those you love how much you
    appreciate them

solve a math problem

speed-read

practice new ways to tie your scarf

create natural dyes from common plants

make caramel from sweetened
    condensed milk

pretend to be a great chef while you are
    cooking

design jewelry

practice being foppish

play with a yo-yo

do word association exercises

plant a giving tree

sort LEGOs by color

look through binoculars

wax and press leaves

list all the foods you know are yellow

eat some fiber or protein

learn a hog call

take a time-lapse video 📱

create a customized crossword puzzle
  for your partner, providing clues
  that only the two of you could
  know

learn CPR, first aid, and the Heimlich
  maneuver

drive to a park

define a problem you want to solve

decide what to do with the rest of
  your life

refinish a table

cook a fancy meal for yourself

stand in the sun

clean your glasses

make a Thai iced tea

explore a new area in your hometown

register for swimming lessons

check the blind spot

head to a trailhead

attend a brown-bag talk at a college

get permission for something you want
    to do

start a collection of coins, stamps,
    antiques, or anything that strikes
    your fancy

read between the lines

make a cheer-up or get-well-soon basket
    or card for someone

scale an indoor climbing wall

plan a boat you would like to build

shovel the sidewalk

have a cup of tea or coffee

breathe and feel yourself smile

find a hidden talent

make someone's day

keep a daily journal of your relationship
    with your child

learn 100 basic words in sign language

design a children's toy

pick a letter of the alphabet and base
    your day's activities on it

make an animal friend

buy yourself a present

ask a colleague for advice

pitch a tent

fake an accent

cheer up a melancholy friend

stir-fry food

remove the storm windows

make friends with an elderly neighbor

personalize your cubicle

buy your first ice cream cone of
    the season

replicate Big Mac sauce

get a broader perspective on a situation
    in your life

discover beauty

find the colors that are unique in an
    otherwise monochromatic landscape

identify constellations

feel the coolness of a rock

try a standing backbend

sing all the old camp songs

unpack the last box

rediscover favorite books from
    childhood

visualize a favorite place

take mom and dad out for dinner

pretend the hallway has stairs

make a checklist for something—
    or everything

go for a hike wherever you are

admit someone was right all along

dance whenever the spirit moves you

create a coupon booklet of special favors
    as a gift for someone

develop an understanding of the natural world

draw escape maps

taste and adjust the seasoning of a dish

time yourself in an activity and then keep trying to beat your time

look at all the details of a leaf in the sunshine

trail an ant

motivate someone through a tough task

shell peas

open a window or door to bring in fresh air

lay a stick trail in the woods

go to a college and sit in on different classes

gather firewood

donate groceries to a local food bank

admire an old building

double-dig a flower bed

**hold deep discussions with
  your pet**

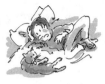

sift flour

learn to do a headstand

clean out the place or room that needs it
  the most

drag your partner on boring errands to
  make them more fun

try 3D drawing

fit one more book on the bookshelf

put dead plants in compost bins

read a book you normally wouldn't
  pick up

research a topic that has been nagging
  at you

clean out and organize your wallet

bag litter when you go on a walk

come up with a great idea

envisage the far future

do lunges

make a checking account deposit

write down all the different roles
you play

take a brisk walk around the block

look for *an* answer instead of *the* answer

figure out your favorite smell and seek
it out

do a common thing in an uncommon way

take an aromatherapy bath

give anonymously to charity

set up a breakfast tray the night before

savor the moment and its impermanence

put together a hiking backpack so you're
ready to go any time

name all your daily routines

put old catalogs in the recycling bin

put lotion on your feet and then pull on
a pair of socks for a moisturizing
treatment

prepare a bad day survival kit full of things that give you joy

slide down a banister

improve your communication skills

try salt painting

get to know every painting in your favorite museum

donate puzzle books to hospitals

focus on just one thing, even if it does not appeal, and train yourself to be open to an unexpected, delightful discovery

tear a page off a calendar so today's date shows

fix a broken family heirloom

bring back to mind an idea you've forgotten and allow it to ripen

design your own invitation

ask an outrageous question

count the number of animal feet you see in one minute

place and tend an edible plant in your
  backyard

tend to an orchid

put address labels in your notebooks

act out a fantasy

discuss summer vacation plans

sit outside during a spring storm

watch baseball from the bleachers

make window cleaner using vinegar and
  water with a drop of liquid soap

make a chalk maze on the driveway

type one-handed

visualize peeling an apple
  in your head

pack someone else's lunch

socialize

allow thinking, but do not engage in your
  thoughts

create a compost area in the yard

attempt a handstand

learn how to do a proper push-up

do quilling, or rolling paper art

watch the gradual creep of shadows

poach fruit

try a food that scares you

commit all seven sins without causing
serious harm

make your bed while you are still in it

simplify household routines

figure out direction by using the sun

write at least 250 words every morning
before going to work

attend to a minor detail that you might
otherwise overlook

do alternate nostril breathing
(pranayama) for 10 rounds

howl at the moon

load the dishwasher

raise awareness of an important issue

put a brand-new screen in a window

atone for a sin

take yourself out on a date

appreciate all that went into a meal

do the dishes right after dinner

repeat a mantra

discover things about your surroundings
you never noticed before

describe a scene in detail

cloister yourself away to do nothing but
write

put in earplugs and enjoy inner peace

empower people by teaching and by
being an example

set something in motion

be sure you know everyone in your office

make a cat or dog toy that looks like your
cat or dog

hike a short trail and then hike it the
opposite direction

load gear into the car

dance without music

complete a tidying project

peel vegetables

draw and paint under a tree

evaluate all your miscellaneous items,
keeping only things you love

create poems based on the titles of books

play softball

outline a novel

enjoy a hot drink in the park

patiently watch a bud open

tie up loose ends

do something for which silence is
required

rediscover card games, board games, and
the outdoors

build a cat tree for your cat

bring breakfast fixings over to a friend's
house and cook something together

listen to the sounds around you and
when one grabs your attention,
dwell on it

mind-map your ideas

plan a visit to a farm

talk to a stuffed animal

squeegee the windows

pretend you are a secret agent

scan crowds for people of interest

play a child's favorite game

bless a sneezer

have a Chinese takeout party

achieve a perfect lotus pose in yoga

find a great book to use as a resource

harmonize on a song

organize a bag of necessities to keep in
your car trunk

toss a grape and catch it in your mouth

make a car for the Soap Box Derby

practice stream-of-consciousness writing

take a breather

thank someone

make the dinner salad

spend part of your workday pursuing speculative new ideas

make up a cheer with the letters of your best friend's name

bunny-hop a bike

create a clubhouse

build castles in the air for fun

find your grandmother's recipe for a favorite food

paint a design on a T-shirt

explore a cave

notice the change in the feeling of cat fur as it gets a little softer at the jawline

discover a new hobby

go for a five-mile walk before breakfast

complete a challenge

perfect a foreign accent

change your hair part

admire yourself

josh around with your colleagues

call your representatives and make your opinion heard

visit a historical monument or tourist attraction

remove scuffs from hardwood floors

do driving therapy, where thoughts get a chance to grow or lapse

browse a dictionary

return stray tools to the toolbox

attempt what you've always wondered about

exchange smiles

wash winter sweaters

stroke the mossy bark of a tree

eat fast food slowly

indulge a child

sidewalk surf on a skateboard

display an objet d'art

examine any subject that arouses
    curiosity

make a campaign contribution

sharpen all your pencils

learn to cook real fried chicken

allow sleep to wrap you in its muffling
    layers

do a cartwheel

bike down a remote trail

change the baking soda in the
    refrigerator and freezer

paint miniatures

emulate a role model

remember to bring your phone charger

take in the scent of toast toasting

make a constructive criticism

learn the art of field sketching

curl up with a book in front of a fireplace

help a child in need

do a visualization exercise

explore the beach at low tide

read with someone you love

reward a child for doing a good deed

solve an acrostic

patch things up with a friend

draw what you see

pretreat a stain before washing

stack kindling in neat piles

be hospitable

play checkers

place a cool or warm washcloth
on your eyes

celebrate new holidays

get rid of attic junk

take a moment to be aware of the smells,
textures, and noises around you

interrupt someone's yawn

go to a children's museum

jazz up fabric sneakers

look at all the colors you can see on
a cloudy day

separate your garbage from recyclable
items

make a call you've been dreading

beachcomb

find lost treasure in the bottom of your
dresser drawers

arrange dried flowers

dawdle at every store window

make drink coasters

ask yourself, "What if?"

straighten the pantry

visit a nearby open house

create a clear sense-memory of a positive
mental state

snoop around the basement

look for an answer

list your favorite candies in order

show up

compost your food waste for a worm
farm

apologize

improve the quality of your day

begin the day by saying, "I am awake and
grateful to be alive"

seesaw at the park

try new healthy recipes

snuggle under a blanket when it is chilly

cut flowers and place them in a vase,
looking closely at the petals, colors,
and leaves

pass a note without getting caught

show someone the ropes

dangle your feet in water

jump over waves

deep-six a bad idea

decide on a fun sideline project

notice and deeply enjoy every sip or bite

do a wacky science experiment

gather friends

learn how to bind a book from scratch 📱

drive down roads with rewarding landscapes

plan a birthday celebration

repair a window screen

make a cake for someone

count shooting stars

take a book or newspaper to dinner when you are alone

gambol and cavort

keep a curiosity file

show respect

design a children's playground

slam-dunk a doughnut

work on a book

prepare your favorite snack food

try to do nothing

learn how to breathe properly when running or singing

take your glasses off and rest your eyes

find the center and the exit of a maze

finish a big school project

feel the cool wind on your face when you bike

find an interesting backdrop and wait for a compelling subject to wander into it

photograph street art

sit alone with your own thoughts

poke a fire

enjoy the excitement of a crowd

hang the laundry outside to dry

draw a favorite room in your childhood home, including every detail you can remember raise sunflowers

decorate a card's envelope

draw half of a picture and ask someone
    else to finish it

invest your money

enjoy some quality one-on-one time with
    your pet

do holiday decorating with lots of funny
    items

mold gelatin

send a letter to your old address,
    describing a memory of living there

label packages in the refrigerator and
    freezer

host a friends-of-friends party

leave 15 minutes earlier than you think
    you must to reach a destination

visit a haunted house

have tea and crumpets

hang clothes that look like they would be
    happier hung up

play Trivial Pursuit

make a Buddha statue out
of stones in your yard

crack the whip to get a project done

splash acrylic paint onto a canvas

read a book you've been wanting to read
forever

reveal your deepest secret to your
closest friend

clean out all those little drawers in
the bathroom

guess a person's occupation

go to the grocery store and buy the
products you might run out of soon

practice cobra pose

invent a cure for your own cold

be with others with no need to fill
the silence

create a character from scratch,
beginning with their name

make your own whipped cream

draw shadows

create your own art style that you can then perfect

break bread with family

create "best of" lists at the end of the year

volunteer time at an animal shelter

have a checklist ready for any type of trip or event

identify everyone in old family photographs

look for a good luck penny on the ground

adjectivize words

learn power walking for fitness

be happily alone in a crowd

go sledding in a snow saucer

grow herbs in a window garden

watch fog blown inland from the sea

collage a cigar box

play tennis

dust behind the furniture

cultivate an ant farm

daydream, which demands something of
you and feeds inner life

teach someone how to be kind

rescue an earthworm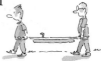

learn Morse code

try a recipe with aquafaba, the flavorless,
whippable water in canned beans

count each step of a walk

examine the texture of your throw pillows

track everything you spend for a week

observe the effect that certain foods have
on you

rake leaves

get that pesky facial hair with tweezers

wax a car

say something positive

turn your attention from dissatisfaction
to gratitude

dillydally

put a bow on your pet

learn to cook Cajun style

go on a controlled shopping spree

do a mindful body scan, either in a chair
or lying down

play volleyball

open a book at random and read for
a short while

interrupt your daily routine to do
something out of the ordinary

close your eyes and breathe in deeply

wash your hair

check out a new or unusual store

stack books by the bed in the order you
want to read them

nurture a living thing

rinse out the sink

catch sight of the setting sun

attempt something of your choice for a
day to see what it is like—carpe diem!

listen to a splashing fountain

write a fan letter to your favorite living
author

make home fries

watch a bird in flight for as long as
you can

ride your bike

do something creative

walk aimlessly

build a campfire

make a bowl from an old 33 rpm
record

pay close attention to a stranger

take a big hard book to a big soft chair

stuff gloves into pockets

explore yourself through lists

join a book group

blow a kiss

create an elaborate hopscotch course

label your power cords

choose a Christmas craft project

eat chocolate

devote time to seeing a
new painting

collect rainwater

serve a meal of all
bite-size portions

create a cartoon

do brainteasers

feed the dog under the table

explore your own backyard

examine nature's designs

lift weights

beat the rugs

comfort someone afflicted with sorrow

place an order at the deli

overcome writer's block

discover the origin of your name

start out someone's day with a joke or
funny story

rediscover an interest or hobby

nurture others' creativity

offer nourishment

help one person

pray

propagate houseplants from cuttings

smile until you feel it

observe vehicles around you

pick a great location to watch the sun
come up or go down

make a date with friends to watch the
next meteor shower

make a birdbath

do undone tasks by candlelight

make an Advent calendar

survey life from a rooftop

gently remove an insect
from your home

jam with friends

talk with Morse code using a flashlight

paint rocks

peel off a jar or bottle label

do the dishes for someone

return all your phone calls

remodel a room on paper

go to a bowling alley

venture into the wilderness

do chair-based exercises

map favorite foods in your area

help with yard work

alternate normal walking with short
    sprints

look at a map upside down

paint outside

envision how you want something to go
    at school, work, or a special event

look for a small way to improve your
    work

sightsee

play beach volleyball

make words from Alpha-Bits cereal or
   alphabet pasta

do hand exercises to prevent or relieve
   carpal tunnel syndrome

come up with a family motto

take twice as much time
   as usual to eat

enroll in an art class

separate egg whites from yolks

read Proust

forage for food in the wilderness

challenge an assumption

walk around a lake

make a big pot of soup

find ways to maximize battery life 📱

spend time with your pet as part of your
   transition from work to home

imagine your current scene as a
   photograph

go bouldering at a gym

throw all the dirty clothes in the hamper or washing machine

summarize the day in one poetic sentence

play jacks

dry your hair in the sun or wind

change focus between near and far to expand your perception and enliven your eyes

ask a child to sing you a song

cuddle your child

learn local history

allow everything to be just as it is

"calligraphize" your handwriting

grind your own coffee beans

forecast the weather

create a business plan for starting your own company

outline a term or work paper

learn how to box out in basketball

create beauty

watch the flight of shorebirds

tidy a cupboard

try a different pizza topping

dust everywhere you have avoided
dusting

make your bed

place reading glasses in strategic spots in
the house

figure out a world record you want to
attempt

splatter paint

ramble down a country lane

play on an adult exercise playground

rehearse a task mentally

rappel down a climbing gym's wall

donate supplies or food to the local
animal shelter or animal rescue
group

practice mountain pose

eavesdrop while waiting in line

decide not to worry about a recent disagreement

make a big decision

pop Goldfish crackers

take a battery of tests to identify your strengths and weaknesses

peel a grape

bring together two great ideas

bake two dozen cookies and drop them off at the firehouse

cook a new combo of veggies

be here, not elsewhere

do a Barbie's hair

have a picnic in bed

put out a can so you can measure the rain

find a good climbing tree

think about something you know nothing about, then explore it

sit up, lean forward, ask questions, and
    nod your head

center a picture on the wall

refinish a piece of furniture

paint a concrete sidewalk to look like
    a brick path

wade in a creek

notice a cat taking a deep sigh before
    starting a nap

outline a big project

ice-skate

go for a family bike ride

pay a toll for someone

become enmeshed with an idea you are
    developing

learn to cook

make cupcakes

do a self-care activity

send compliments to the chef

change the artwork on your walls

contemplate the colors on a map

use unneeded food storage containers for organizing things in drawers

cook on an outdoor grill in midwinter

notice some feeling within you and identify the source of that feeling

imagine the world from your pet's point of view

make a basic cat's cradle with two yards of string

annoy someone and thoroughly enjoy it

prepare soil for the garden

pretend your car is an airplane or spaceship

get rid of all broken appliances

be curious about what is happening in your body

chat over tea, coffee, or hot chocolate

scavenge for materials that can be used for your projects

go in early to the office

give comfort to others

measure spaghetti

blend fresh juices

swap lunches

hold forth with a group of people

head south

walk in the snow at night

create a budget that you can stick to

change someone's mind for the better

let yourself rest

tiptoe on a creaky floor

answer children's letters to Santa Claus

spot a security camera and point at it

gather all the papers in your house in
    one place

melt old crayons into an art project

fertilize your vocabulary

increase yin by doing stretching
    exercises like yoga and tai chi

put potato chips on a sandwich for crunch

get a baton or drumstick and twirl it

deodorize the litter box

find the burned-out bulb on a string of
    Christmas tree lights

color an entire coloring book

feel the cool evening breeze as it
    dissipates the summer heat

peel potatoes

exorcise your demons

make a balloon dog

declutter a particularly busy area of your
    home

start a brand-new notebook

taste autumn in an apple

plan a big celebration

leave a happy message under car
    windshield wipers

clean out a drawer

keep a commonplace book with passages, poetry, and quotes that you want to remember

rearrange knickknacks

design a bridge

pre-soften butter

leave heads-up pennies for others to find

sketch one thing

read a book of quotations

add color to your life

educate someone

devour a book in one sitting

devise your own method of speed-writing

change an incandescent light bulb to an energy-saving bulb

ease a burden

find little treasures on the ground

chew each bite of food at least 30 times

daydream through your commute

rejuvenate your skin

pack every drawer like a Japanese Bento
box

pull from your past and tinker with
old ideas

call or visit your oldest relative

break up shelves full of books with a few
objects, pictures, and horizontal
stacks

study

create elaborate paintings or new worlds
in your mind

drive along a few back roads

wash someone's hair

make earrings

collect recyclables at the beach

make a balloon bouquet for someone

rescue an unfinished project

take a bag of deposit bottles to the store
to get the cash

foster an injured animal

listen to a dog lap up water

decipher someone's poor handwriting

put a bay leaf under your pillow to see if
it brings sweet dreams

notice the heat, texture, and fragrance of
whatever you're eating

go on a comfort food restaurant tour

consider what message you'd sky-write

write a children's book with the
central character being a child
you know

alter clothing

watch a bird build its nest

do something completely backward or
out of sequence

write lyrics for a song

build a birdhouse

use no words, only signs and gestures

do Walter Camp's Daily Dozen exercise
regimen

scrub mildew off the fence or outdoor
furniture

create a box of memories for a friend

refinish castoffs and turn them into
treasures

make deviled eggs

flip a coin

spot for someone who is bench-pressing

chant a mantra

piece together the shards of a pot

throw yourself a party

cheer someone on

go to a book signing

open every window in the house

pick out tomorrow's outfit

give every friend a silly nickname

look for a feather on the beach

enjoy quiet moments removing the snow, one shovelful at a time

conquer a fear

make a baby laugh by making funny sounds

do a backpacking meditation

donate food to a hunger program

finish something

put gloves in the glove compartment

pay all your bills

practice chopping like a chef

look at a handful of sand closely

draw abstract designs without lifting the pen off the paper

replenish your wish list

learn archery

lead a club or group activity

declare open season on something, such as rude behavior

put appreciation into words

set your intention for the day

take a nap on the beach

tour a new town

concoct someone's favorite beverage

cuddle

take over a chore that your spouse
    dreads

mix colors on a palette

maintain a car's finish

learn how to bait a fishhook

investigate an archaeological site in
    your hometown

do laundry mindfully

garden

appreciate everything that feels good
    about your body

brew a pot of tea

notice that you cannot think and
    be aware of your breathing at the
    same time

find beauty hiding in the ordinary

breathe life into an old project

climb to a lookout point

look for an idea in a strange, unexpected place

design clothes

look at your schedule and make time to volunteer

read *National Geographic* in a waiting room

make a seven-letter word in Scrabble

learn CB (citizens band) lingo

have a beach party indoors

find a four-leaf clover

do a backspin serve in table tennis

make book covers out of brown paper bags

sample a simpler life

annotate your favorite book

take and lift fingerprints

navel gaze

dance around in your underwear

sculpt ribbons to decorate packages

go bowling

belt out a torch song

put fresh pepper in the shaker

make sun tea

identify something by touch

seek inner peace

read four pages of a print dictionary

research your options for something you
don't know how to proceed on

create a bingo game

learn to be ambidextrous

tweeze chin whiskers

navigate by the stars

hide money in someone's pocket

conceptualize a new car design

balance the checkbook

ask parents about the good old days

list pros and cons before making a big
    decision

display your most cherished possession

choose a poem to bring with you
    wherever you go

match all the socks

list your favorite smells

make a 3D model of a building

inventory the house

take a 10-minute vacation

surrender to a hammock or lounge chair

meditate during a staff meeting

put spare change in a charity bucket

schedule time to play with children

think up a bumper sticker slogan

gad about town

switch to more comfortable clothes

wink at random passersby

find serenity

trek to a planetarium

hypnotize someone

replace something worn out

write with both hands at once

detail a car

shinny up a tree

fend off a snack attack

winterize your home

choose your own path

find two friends and do the limbo

draw patterns that repeat

form a knitting group

rejuvenate an old fruit tree

network at an event

time yourself counting to a thousand

grow lettuce hydroponically

earthquake-proof your house

mold clay

allow feelings to come and go

trace an intricate pattern

stare off into the middle distance

straighten up the house

make a 30-day waiting list for things you want to buy

do now what you keep saying you ought to do someday

watch squirrels cross a road

make a *big* plan

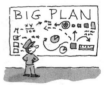

go onstage on amateur night at a local comedy club

appreciate something that annoys you

make prolonged eye contact with everyone you meet

yodel in the stairwell

curate your memory

do leaf and bark rubbings of trees in the yard

join a bird walk at a nature center

pick a flower for someone

read a book chapter out loud in an accent

create a beautiful fan for a hot summer day

start a list of 1,001 things

have a make-your-own-sundae party

look at a comic book

find a book you have been searching for

watch a baby fall asleep

learn how an everyday object, like a clock, works

write the Greek alphabet

make a bow and arrow

paint a bird's-eye view

be audaciously present

ACKNOWLEDGMENTS

Thank you to the idea-maker behind this book, my editor, Mary Ellen O'Neill. Thank you, too, to the editorial team of Anna Cooperberg and Susan Bolotin; production editor Dylan Julian; designer Galen Smith; and illustrator Scot Ritchie for the brilliant drawings. I will be eternally grateful to the idea-maker behind this company, Peter Workman. I feel lucky to have been a Workman author for 30 years.

ABOUT THE AUTHOR

Author of the bestseller *14,000 Things to Be Happy About*, **Barbara Ann Kipfer** has written more than 80 books and calendars of wit and inspiration, thesauri and dictionaries, trivia and question books, archaeology reference books, and happiness and spiritually themed books. Kipfer is a professional lexicographer and holds PhDs in Linguistics, Archaeology, and Buddhist Studies.